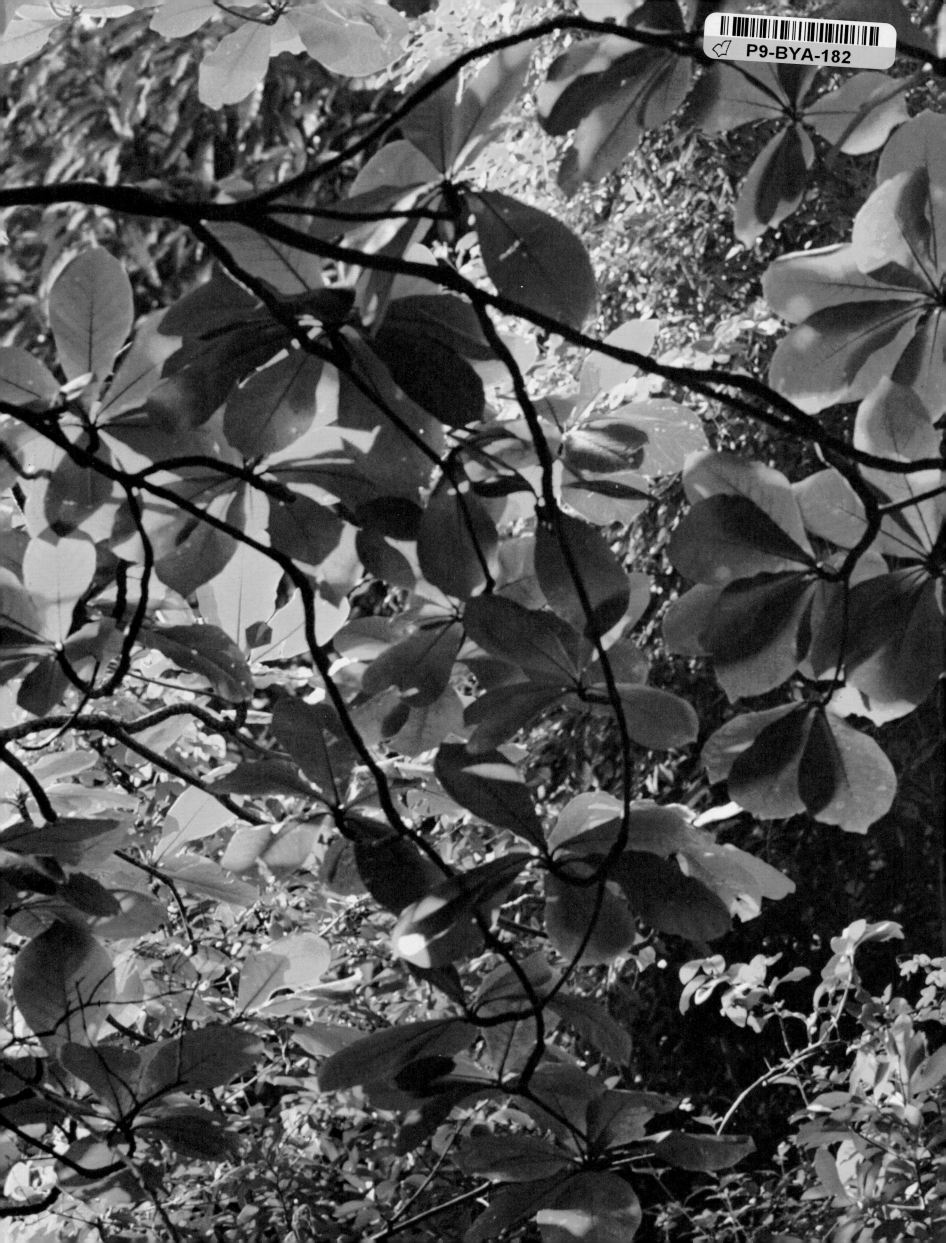

P9-BYA-182

IN THE SAME ORIGINAL FORMAT, GENERAL EDITOR AND DESIGNER DAVID BROWER:

This Is the American Earth, by Ansel Adams and Nancy Newhall

Words of the Earth, by Cedric Wright

These We Inherit: The Parklands of America, by Ansel Adams

"In Wildness Is the Preservation of the World," by Eliot Porter

The Place No One Knew: Glen Canyon on the Colorado, by Eliot Porter

The Last Redwoods: Photographs and Story of a Vanishing Scenic Resource, by
    Philip Hyde and Francois Leydet

Ansel Adams: A Biography. Volume I: The Eloquent Light, by Nancy Newhall

Time and the River Flowing: Grand Canyon, by Francois Leydet

Gentle Wilderness: The Sierra Nevada, text from John Muir,
    photographs by Richard Kauffman

Not Man Apart: Photographs of the Big Sur Coast,
    with lines from Robinson Jeffers

The Wild Cascades: Forgotten Parkland, by Harvey Manning,
    with lines from Theodore Roethke

Everest: The West Ridge, by Thomas F. Hornbein, with
    photographs from the American Mount Everest Expedition

Summer Island: Penobscot Country, by Eliot Porter

Navajo Wildlands: As Long as the Rivers Shall Run, photographs by
    Philip Hyde, text by Stephen Jett, edited by Kenneth Brower

Kauai and the Park Country of Hawaii, by Robert Wenkam
    edited by Kenneth Brower

Glacier Bay: The Land and the Silence, by Dave Bohn

Baja California and the Geography of Hope, photographs by Eliot Porter,
    text by Joseph Wood Krutch, edited by Kenneth Brower

Central Park Country: A Tune Within Us, photographs by Nancy and Retta
    Johnston, text by Mireille Johnston, introduction by Marianne Moore

Galapagos: The Flower of Wildness (both volumes edited by Kenneth Brower)

1. *Discovery*, photographs by Eliot Porter, introduction by Loren Eiseley,
    with selections from Charles Darwin, Herman Melville, and others; and

2. *Prospect*, photographs by Eliot Porter, introduction by John P. Milton,
    text by Eliot Porter and Kenneth Brower

THE EARTH'S WILD PLACES

Maui: The Last Hawaiian Place, by Robert Wenkam,
    edited, with Kipahulu Sketches, by Kenneth Brower

Return to the Alps, by Max Knight and Gerhard Klammet,
    edited, with selections from Alpine literature, by David R. Brower

The Primal Alliance, Earth and Ocean, by John Hay and Richard Kauffman,
    edited by Kenneth Brower

Earth and the Great Weather: The Brooks Range, by Kenneth Brower

Eryri, the Mountains of Longing, by Amory Lovins,
    with photographs by Philip Evans, edited by David R. Brower

A Sense of Place: The Artist and the American Land, by Alan Gussow,
    with illustrations by fifty-nine painters, and foreword by Richard Wilbur

Micronesia: Island Wilderness, by Kenneth Brower and Robert Wenkam

Guale, the Golden Coast of Georgia, James P. Valentine, Robert Hanie,
    Eugene Odom, John P. Milton *et al.*, edited by Kenneth Brower

To Joan, Robert John and Family
June 1976
We hope the recollections of this trip
will bring pleasant memories always.
Myra and Boy.

1.

THE EARTH'S WILD PLACES®
A Friends of the Earth Series

MAUI: The Last Hawaiian Place

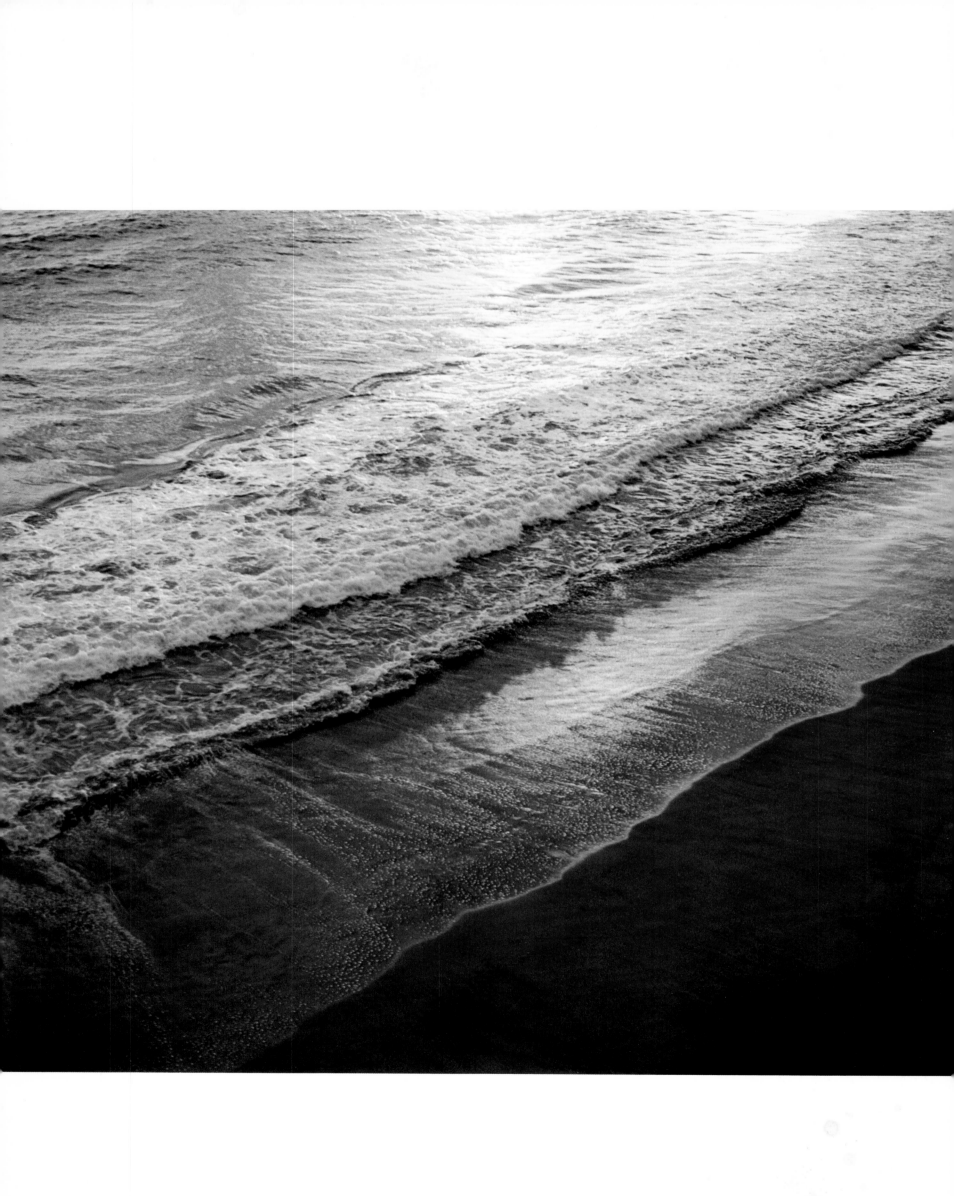

[Hawaii, 1867]

Fishing was one of the chief occupations in old days. The fishhooks were
made of turtle shell, dog, fish or human bones, prongs of hard wood, and
other materials. Fish were caught in deep-sea fishing grounds of a depth of from
thirty to forty fathoms, or sometimes of four hundred fathoms . . .
Fishermen went in search of such fishing grounds and learned to locate
a particular spot and to return to it again and again. They kept its location a
secret from others; it was like a food dish to them. Today the knowledge
of most of these places is lost.

. . .

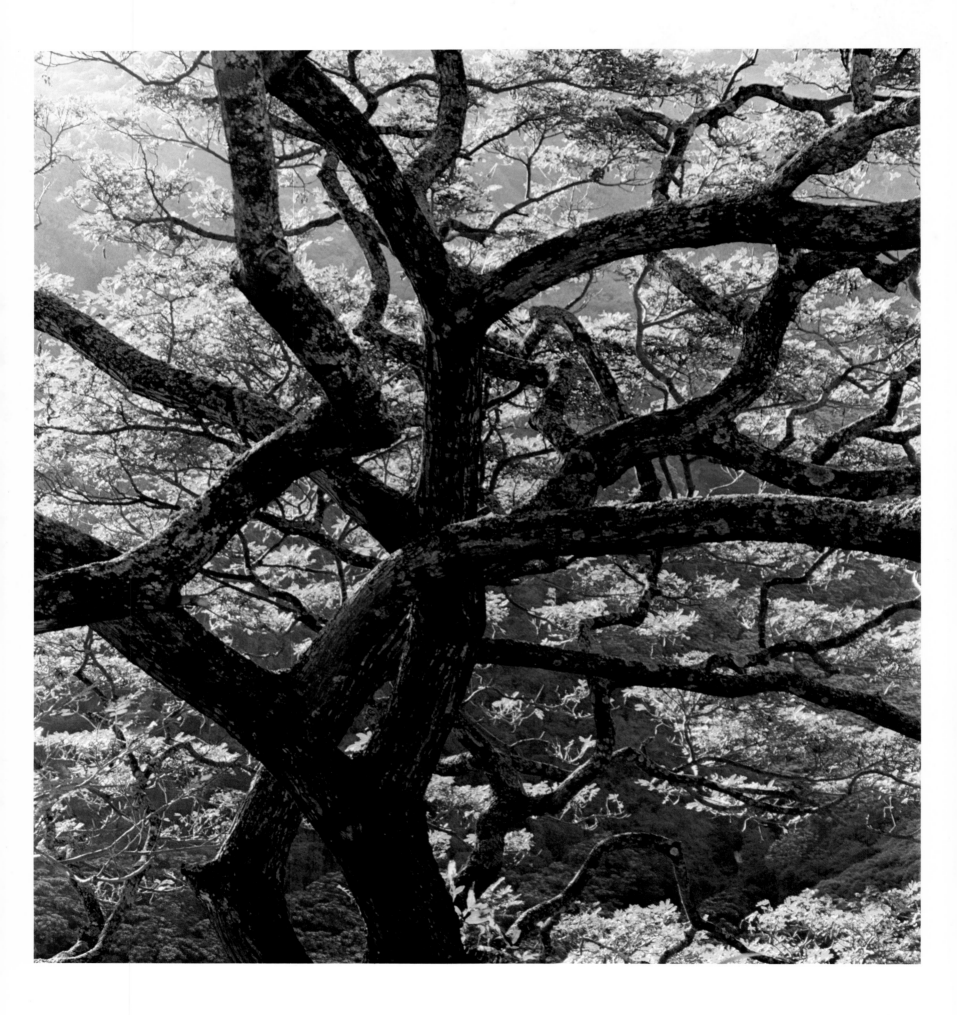

Canoe-making was also an expert art. A canoe kahuna must first own adzes, and these were not of iron but of stone. The best stone for the purpose was the *hokele* rock, the blue lava (*'ala'makahinu*), and the *pahoa*, and the adzes were fashioned at the crater of Pele where the *hokele* rock was to be found; at Kaluako'i on Molokai; and at other places. The finishing was done with an adze called *pupu'ole*, holes were drilled with a shell called *makoloa*, and smaller holes for sewing the planks together with a *makilihoahoa* shell; another instrument for boring holes was fashioned from a dog's bone. To see the tools these people used you would wonder how, with such crude implements, they could fashion a canoe. I have been told by Ka-uhi and Kahi-poleau who sailed on the war canoe of Pele-io-holani that his double war canoe, named Kaneaiai, and said to have been made of planks sewed together, could hold 160 men. Canoes of various kinds were used to travel from island to island for war expeditions, double (*kaulua*) and single (*kaukahi*) canoes, the *peleleu*, and the *hoapipi*. We today could not make some of these things.

. . .

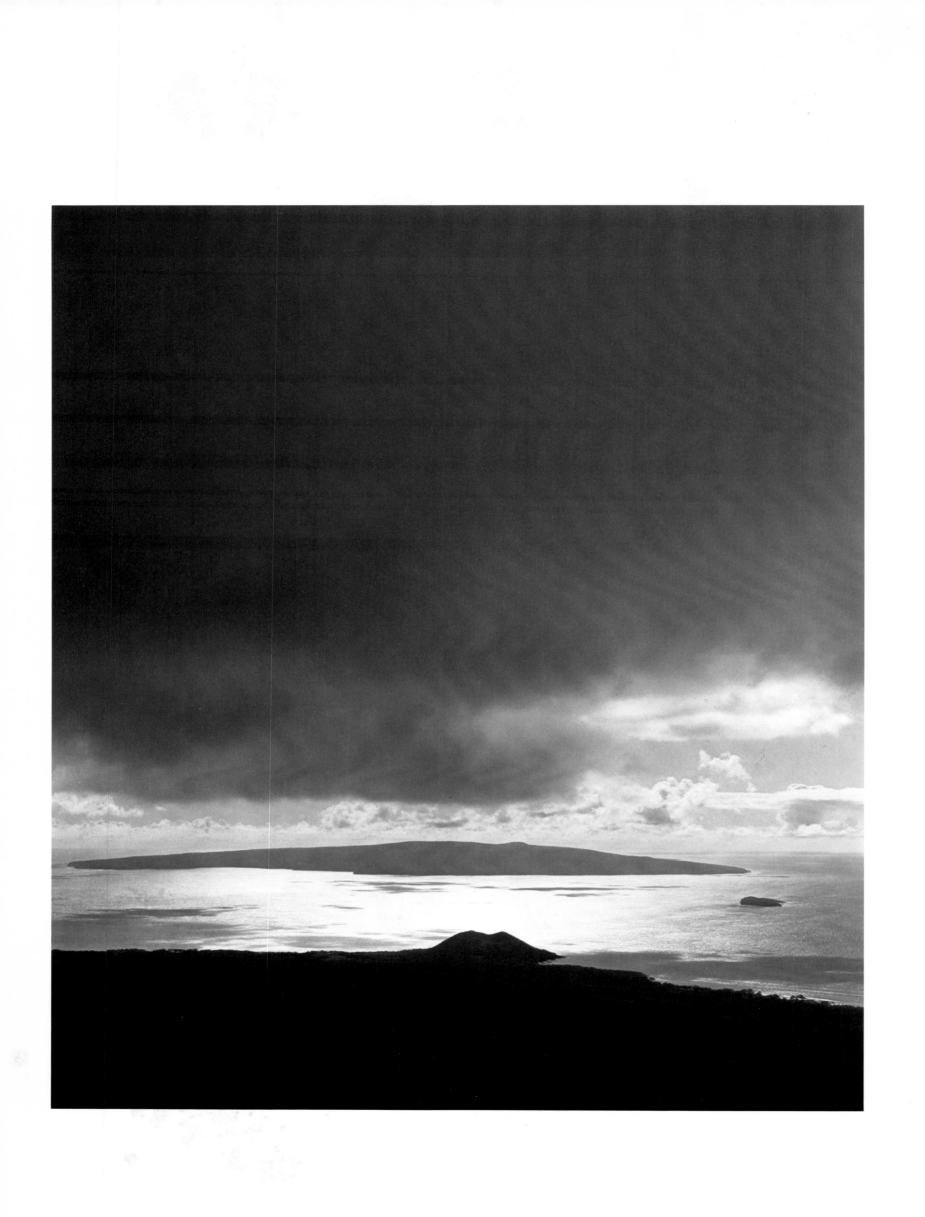

The composing of meles was a skilled art in old days in which some people became famous. They composed chants about the sky, space, the ocean, the earth, sun, moon, stars, and all things. Many had secret meanings woven into them. They were composed of symbolic phrases (*loina*) and hidden meanings (*kaona*). There were many kinds of chant. There were chants in honor of ancestors (*mele kupuna*), in praise of a land (*mele 'aina*), in praise of chiefs (*mele ali'i*), in praise of favorite children (*mele hi'ilani*), chants of gratitude (*mele mahalo*), chants of affection (*mele aloha*), chants of reviling (*kuamuamu*), prayer chants (*mele pule*), dirges (*kanikau*), chants to put a person to sleep (*mele hiamoe*), or to awaken one (*mele ho'ala*), chants asking a favor (*mele noi*), chants refusing the request (*mele 'au'a*), chants calling to be admitted (*mele kahea*), chants given as a gift (*mele haawi*), chants of boasting (*mele ho'oki'eki'e*), prophetic chants (*mele wanana*), chants foretelling future events (*mele kilokilo*), chants of criticism (*mele nemanema*).

. . .

Some of these chants are of great value, some are worthless. Chants uttered in monotone (*olioli*) are prayer chants, but they are not all uttered alike.
The tone is softened (*aheahe*) in places and forced from the throat ('*i*'*i ikaika*).
Some are uttered with a sonorous (*nonolo*) sound, a gurgling ('*ola*'*ola*'), the chanter breathing all the while gently with a gentle rise and fall of the chest.
Each word must be well uttered by the tongue with the mouth open and the teeth separate, and the mouth opened and closed without tightening the neck muscles. The ancients were excellent chanters.

    In the recitation of a genealogy (*ko*'*ihonua*) the voice took a tone almost on one note (*kamakua*), and each word was enunciated distinctly. There was a vibration (*kuolo*) in the chanting together with a guttural sound (*kaohi*) in the throat and a gurgling (*alala*) in the voice box. The voice was to be brought out with strength (*haanou*) and so held in control (*kohi*) that every word was clear. The genealogical chant recited the ancestry of chiefs, their rank and lineage, from a period long before the peopling of Hawaii.

. . .

The composers of genealogical chants such as the *ko'ihonua, ha'ikupuna*, and *kamakua*, were men learned in the art who knew the family lines and were skilled in oratory and state-craft. Such chants were composed under tabu. Chants of prophecy and prayer were composed under the inspiration of a spirit. Chants in praise of a name, a favorite child, chants of gratitude, dirges, and many others might be composed by any person and completed in a short time. Each word had to be studied for its meaning, whether lucky or unlucky, and for its effect (in this particular connection), whether it suggested good or bad luck, a stingy or a kind person, a grumbler or a brave one. If a group worked together to compose a chant the leader would ask each composer to give a line; if there were eighty composers the chant would contain eighty lines, and these would be combined into a single composition. Two, three, or more composers could work on a single chant. The chants were skillfully composed and very pleasing and well fitted to the characteristics of the person for whom each was composed. Generally such chants were composed for chiefs, or by parents for their own children, or for favorite children. Most of them were good but some were licentious in character. The chant might be delightful on the surface, but might have a hidden meaning suggesting stinginess, a refusal to give, or anything else. Most would not catch this meaning and would only see the pleasing picture.

· · ·

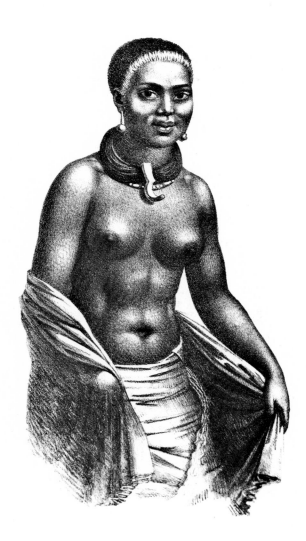

In old days the daughters were made much of
by the parents and grandparents and by the people in general.

· · ·

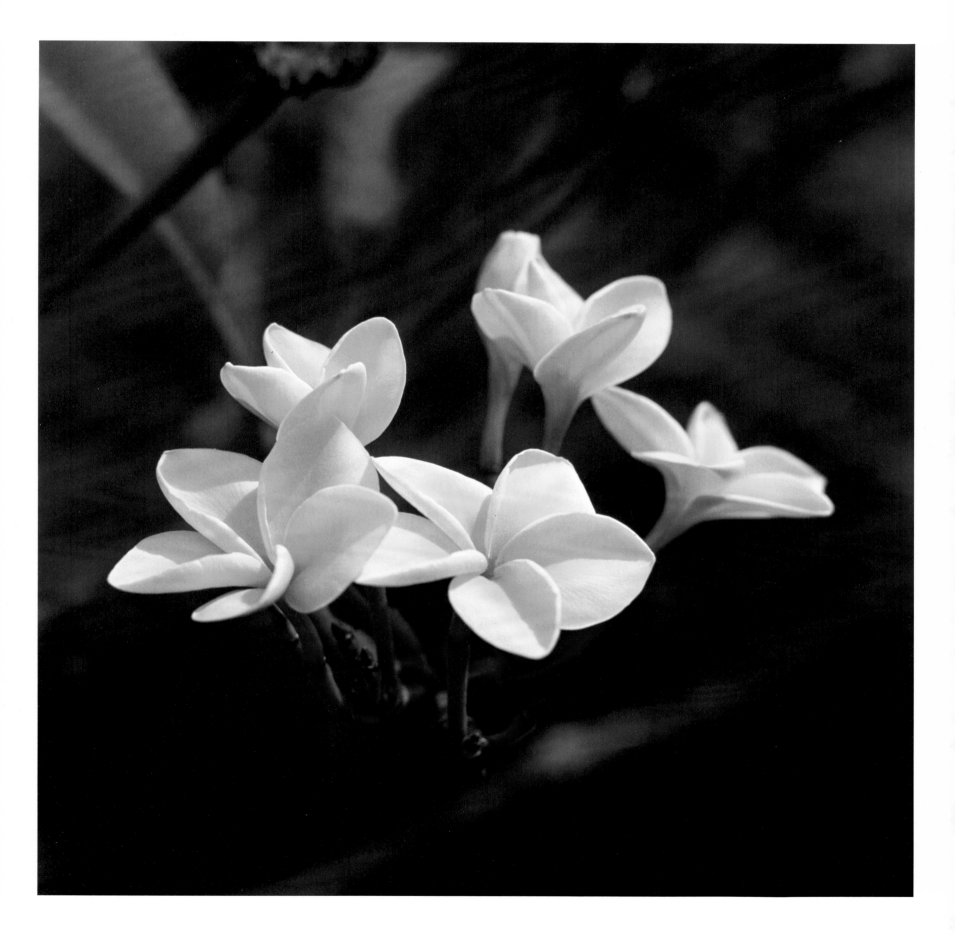

Another ancient art was that of the diviners who revealed hidden things about the land, called "Pointers-out-of-sandhills" (*Kuhikuhi pu'uone*) and "Class of changes on the earth" (*Papahulihonua*). They were able to find things hidden away from the eyes of men; they could locate water in places where water had not been found. They knew the land boundaries from Hawaii to Kauai, the running of the affairs of government, how to handle people, the location and building of houses, and whether one would live or die; they resembled the seers (*kaula*), but there were few such persons in old days and there are none today. Statesmen and orators too have passed away.

—SAMUEL KAMAKAU

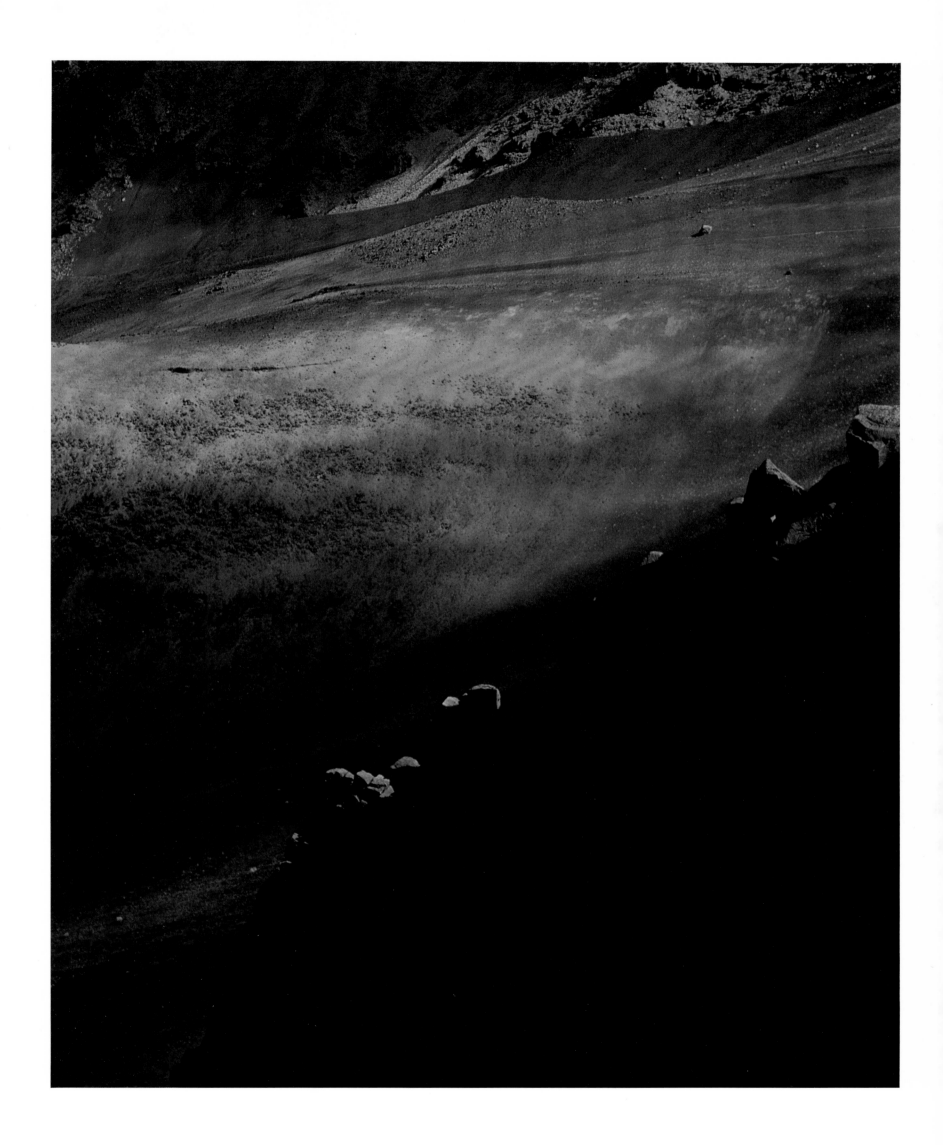

photographs and text by Robert Wenkam

foreword by David R. Brower

introduction by Charles A. Lindbergh

edited, with sketches, by Kenneth Brower

MAUI
The Last Hawaiian Place

FRIENDS OF THE EARTH ✦ SAN FRANCISCO, NEW YORK, LONDON, PARIS
A CONTINUUM BOOK / THE SEABURY PRESS NEW YORK

Silversword, Haleakala

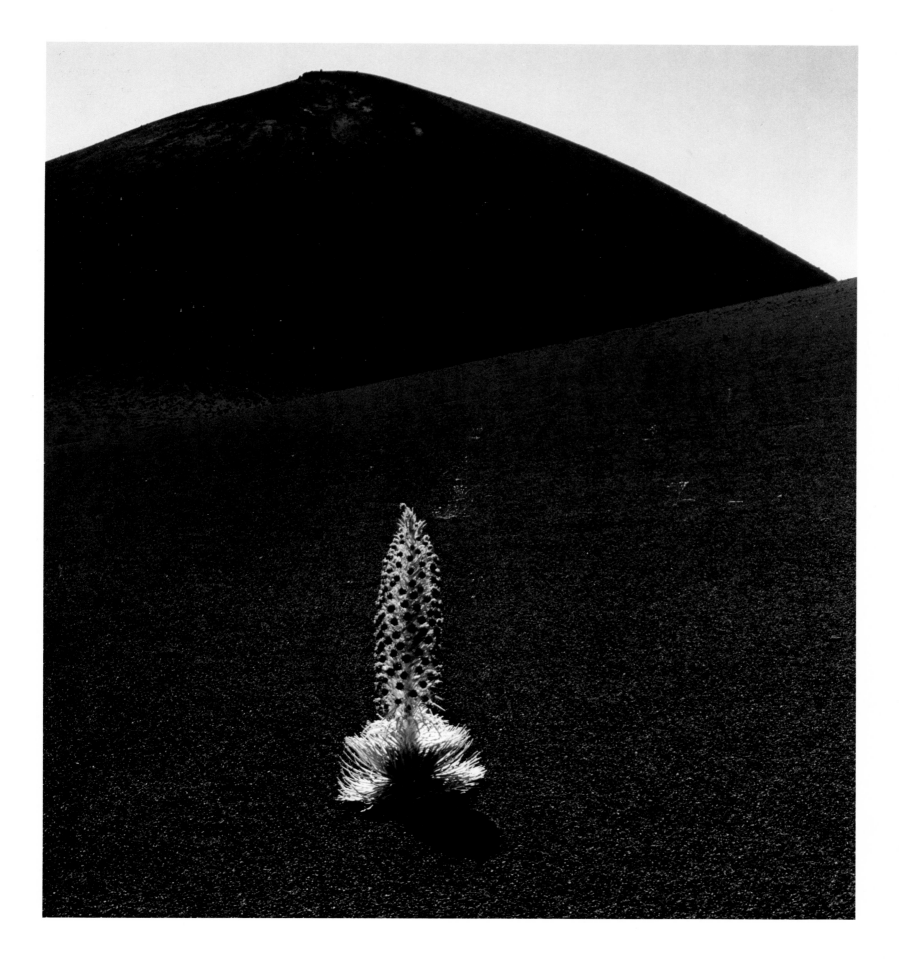

ACKNOWLEDGMENT

The idea for this book began at a hamburger cookout in Kipahulu Valley. Hamilton McCaughey and Huey Johnson were looking at the paperback of my book on Kauai, and asked why I didn't write a book on Maui. Johnson said the book would support the Nature Conservancy's fund drive to buy the Kipahulu land and McCaughey said that wide recognition of East Maui's natural beauty, and its vestige of Hawaiian culture, would be vital to its preservation. They were convinced the project deserved funding, and Johnson, master fund-raiser for the Nature Conservancy, told me how to do it.

Within a month I received the necessary grants and started photography. There were five people who made it possible for me to stop taking advertising photographs of hula girls and spend my time instead on the natural beauty of Kipahulu and Hana: Pardee Erdman of Ulupalakua Ranch, Hamilton McCaughey of Kipahulu Cattle Company, Taylor "Tap" Pryor of Hana Ranch, Laurance Rockefeller, and the Mayor of Maui County, Elmer Cravalho. I am grateful to the Sierra Club Foundation for its assistance, and to the Sierra Club for its participation in the project.

When I needed a place to live in Hana, Nancy and Addison Love gave me the best apartment in their Hana Kai Resort on the shore of Hana Bay. When I needed groceries, Harry Hasegawa of the Hasegawa General Store let me eat now and pay later. I ate well. Sam Pryor lent the four-wheel-drive camper that allowed me to sleep until dawn in remote areas.

The Kahului Branch Library's Hawaiian section is small, but its collection is one of the best in the state. The staff, along with the people at the Wailuku library, were very helpful, especially Janet Sheahan, who came over from the children's room to help with difficult requests, and Mrs. Hilda Voss, Mrs. Lorraine Claytor, Mrs. Ruth Wryn. Regional Librarian Lucille K. Berg graciously allowed me to take her valuable reference copies off the premises to xerox important pages at Mayor Cravalho's office. Especially helpful also were the staffs at the Hawaiian Mission Children's Society Library and at the Hawaiian Sugar Planters' Association Library.

Director Larry Windley of the Lahaina Restoration Foundation lived for a year in Hana and was particularly helpful in following up obscure references and identifying little known people in complex genealogies. Barbara Braasch of *Sunset* magazine was the first to read the completed manuscript and inform me that the book was worthwhile. Karen Paulsen and Hasse Bunnelle helped in polishing up the grammar. Joann Gotsinas, Paula Powell, and Joanne Sheeley typed the manuscript.

Richard Davis, and his outdoor experience, were available whenever I needed them on Maui.

My thanks to Jack Lind and Randy Smith of Kipahulu Cattle Company; Dr. and Mrs. Milton Howell, and John Hanchett of Hana; James Dunn, retired territorial surveyor; Mr. and Mrs. Tokutaro Okada; Chew Kum Chong, retired engineer of the coastal steamer "Makena"; Nick Soon of Kaupo; Rinji Kinoshita, retired owner of Kinoshita Store; Annie Pak Chong and the very charming group of Hawaiian women—all old-time residents—who shared a tape recorder at Kipahulu to talk about the very old days and family genealogies: Mrs. Punihele Haia, Mrs. Annie Smith, Miss Evelyn Cooper, Mrs. Anita (Martinsen) Rockford and Mrs. Daisy (Hussey) McKeabue.

At dinner one evening with Russ Apple, Pacific Historian for the National Park Service, we both found ourselves watching a handsome Hawaiian couple in the Hotel Hana Ranch dining room. I remarked at the regal manner of the husband and wife. Their dress and poise reminded us of the Hawaiian *alii*. We had just that day been exploring Hana's history, and we stared entranced. The Hawaiian across the room had the stature of a Kamehameha, or of a Kiha-a-Piilani, a Hana chief of 400 years ago. Russ could no longer resist asking, walked across the room and introduced himself. The Hawaiian rose, tall and straight, introduced his wife and, unbelievably, said his name was Piilani.

We asked if he would join us the next day in exploring the nearby Piilanihale temple ruins. He agreed and in the morning Russ and I showed a direct descendant of Piilani the temple of his ancestors.

R.W.

We are grateful to the Bernice P. Bishop Museum for permission to print the engravings and the black and white photographs used in this book. (The photograph on page 63 is by Henry C. Ovenden, the photograph on page 90 by L. R. Sullivan.) We are grateful to the Kamehameha Schools Press for permission to reprint excerpts from *Ruling Chiefs of Hawaii*, by Samuel M. Kamakau, copyright 1961.

Copyright in all countries of the International Copyright Union by Friends of the Earth. All rights reserved. Published in New York by Friends of the Earth, Inc., and simultaneously in Paris by Les Amis de la Terre, and in London by Friends of the Earth Ltd.

ISBN 0-913890-04-9

Printed and bound in Italy

This Friends of the Earth/Seabury Press printing contains corrections of minor errors but no substantive changes in text, photographs, or other illustrations. For current information about what is happening in the earth's wild places, write Friends of the Earth, San Francisco.

CONTENTS

FOREWORD, 20

INTRODUCTION, 23

THE LAST HAWAIIAN PLACE,

   Prologue, 26   Origins, 29   Hana, 34

   Kamehameha, 41   Missionaries, 49

   Sugar, 52   The Road, 65   Cattle, 69

   The Park, 78   A Proposal, 89

SOURCES, 92

RAIN SONGS, 96

KIPAHULU SKETCHES, 104

   Herman Nelson, 111   Visitors, 128

   The Linds, 130   William Rost, 144

   The Kaiwis, 147   Pelipe Bernabe, 151

   Nick Soon, 153   The Land, 155

SIXTY-ONE COLOR PLATES

FOREWORD

The best way to remember a place is to go back, and to find it no less than it was. There are still a few places in the Sierra Nevada you can go back to and be pleased how well you remember them and how well wildness cared for them while you were gone. There are probably places on Oahu like this, but La Ronde, overlooking the Ala Moana shopping center and Honolulu, is not one of them. The martinis are good there, and by the time La Ronde has gone full circle you need another. Four years had passed since we last circled there and they had done a great deal of harm. Smog was hanging over Pearl Harbor now, and we could see what Justice William O. Douglas had in mind when, in talking that day to students at the University of Hawaii, he said that real-estate operators are the real planners, that the highway lobby reigns supreme, and that there is an official ecological vandalism abroad that is a combination of public and private greed. A student at one of the informal sessions had remarked, "My father could swim in the Detroit River and I can walk on it." Quite clearly that student could soon walk beyond the beach at Waikiki.

With another martini in hand, I was ready for the next full circle. My recollection of what I saw is probably as accurate as a New Yorker's mental map of the United States, in which the Hudson River lies slightly west of where the Colorado really is: 35 per cent of La Ronde's sweep consisted of shopping center, 10 per cent of high-rise dwellings that obscured the Punchbowl, 10 per cent of high-rise hotels that obliterated the view of Waikiki and another 10 per cent of high-rise structures that had a beach-head on the toe of Diamond Head. Then there was 20 per cent of daggers of development aimed at the heart of Oahu, 5 per cent of smog plume, 2 per cent of Sears Roebuck, 2 per cent of the artificial Magic Island, and 1 per cent of real magic. With but a little more effort, I thought, Hawaii could have another Los Angeles where Honolulu had been. The unaccounted-for 5 per cent slipped by uncatalogued when we overheard a man say, "It was Kaiser who discovered the Hawaiian Islands, not Captain Cook."

Not wanting Mr. Kaiser, Boise-Cascade, or anyone with similar ideas to discover Maui, we remembered hard what we had just been shown there by Robert Wenkam, best of all possible guides to the last Hawaiian place. Maui is symbolic of the islandness of things, and we thought of many coves of beauty that we hoped would never be lessened. We had read some of Kenneth Brower's sketches and wanted to learn about their source directly. In Hana harbor, our first stop after the Maui airport, the spirit informing the people Ken wrote about revealed itself in a moving inscription:

IN MEMORIAM
IN HONOR OF ALL AMERICANS
OF THE HANA DISTRICT
WHO DIED IN THE SERVICE
OF THEIR COUNTRY
THAT BEAUTY AND FREEDOM
OF OUR LAND BE PRESERVED
FOR ALL HUMANITY
1962

To leave a planet in the struggle to keep beauty and freedom alive on it for all humanity is to join "the time-sifted few that leave the world . . . not the same place it was." It is a brave mission because beauty and freedom are dying there. Man can add to the heritage of freedom, however ineptly he sometimes goes about it, but he can hardly add to the wealth of wild beauty that all humanity inherited. He seems able only to diminish it. As we circled Maui we saw how part of that trend might be reversed.

It was no ordinary cocktail hour that ended our first afternoon on Maui. We gathered with friends of Bob Wenkam on the porch of a superbly conceived house built in isolation on Maui's wild east coast. The darkening Pacific was doing all the things an ocean of its experience should be doing when it meets such a coast. As evening began, new drama was added by a squall that moved down on us from the north, scuffing the sea before it. I made a lucky guess that we would have six minutes before the rain would drive us indoors. Until then we could feel it happen—the smell of the air changing as its pace livened and it pressed against us, the subdued wind sound growing more intense, the waves whitening and adding a new tone to the fugue. The first freshening drops fell, and those who were not soakably dressed or who did not want their drinks diluted stepped inside, and I was not the last.

There was man-made beauty indoors to blend nicely with a Mauian beauty that had preceded man on this coast. But was it right, I wondered, that one house, or the two or three that could cluster here in harmony, should have to itself so large a part of one of the most beautiful places of all? Where would that leave all humanity, for whom preserving such beauty was just as important as it was for our friends?

No easy answer came then, nor does it now. Even if

humanity, in an immediate and prolonged exercise of good judgment, should halve its numbers, no single beauty spot could withstand more than a tiny fraction of that half. Some kinds of beauty have to be put in a please-do-not-handle category, with humanity settling for a chance merely to pass by and look, or with being glad to know that such beauty exists, with its community of life enjoying an integrity that can continue only in the absence of predatory man.

Such places need to be known about, lest they be lost by default. They then need to be watched over, and human continuity of knowing about their importance is essential. The antiquities of man have so far been easier to know about than the antiquities of nature, such as the scenic and ecologically important climaxes of Maui, and the National Park System is the safest category yet invented in which to protect them. Haleakala National Park thus preserves the crater. One can drive to two vista points and see the spectacle without footprinting it. Trails make its more intimate details accessible to those who wish to earn the experience by putting to use the nearly universal ability to walk and breathe deep. Regulations about staying on the trails protect the most fragile of places, such as the silversword nurseries. But Haleakala National Park is only half as large as it should be if the park is to represent the wild sweep from crater to the sea that Kipahulu is, and that so much of this book is about. Nor is national park status the ultimate sanctuary. The National Park Service falls victim to the urge to overdevelop (the Forest Service, to overlog) to lure the very people who threaten parks most. The adamant overengineering of the Tioga Road across Yosemite National Park is one of the saddest examples of this weakness. There is, in the end, no substitute for eternal vigilance that recognizes the frailty of the scenic and ecological resources being preserved—the frailty and the irreplaceability of them—and the need to err on the side of preserving too much too carefully if there is to be error at all.

Eternal vigilance, then, by whom? If it is to be by the National Park Service, then we must recognize the great risks entailed in waiting for Congress to recognize the need to establish or expand reserves and for the citizen lobby to overpower the development-and-construction lobby long enough to enable Congress to move. "The American people are light years ahead of Congress in understanding of environmental decline," Justice Douglas told the University of Hawaii audience; but Congress is still light years ahead of the American people in understanding what must be done if a man who takes up political life wants to remain politically alive. National park visi-

tors have not yet, as a body, become very good campaign contributors or doorbell ringers at campaign time, or writers of letters and speeches, or callers at offices or setters up of meetings, or at the making of films and books that altogether can build a constituency. A goal achieved without a constituency is like an overdraft, and as quickly returned to the maker.

The political process must necessarily transcend fad, half-think, and hang-up—yet it is run by people who fall victim to those very ills. While they recover, what can be done to keep Californians and Texans and Boise-Cascadians from buying, subdividing, and forever alienating the best of unspoiled Maui?

Here, I think—and this is what I was trying to work out as I carried my drink in out of the rain—is where latter-day noblemen can perform, and are performing, an indispensable role. It is the same role their ancestors played for three centuries in preserving, for their own reasons, beautiful places and complex ecosystems that would otherwise have been severed from the earth's biological wealth and have been lost, beyond recall. Should we not thank the people of far beyond ordinary means who have cared enough about the beauty of land and of the way it works to hang onto it, to love it, to bring it at no little expense down through their time to our time? Whatever their reasons for achieving what they did, they held a place together and set a style for private conservation. Their role will be needed until society as a whole becomes progressive enough to stop the clock on new development, to declare that whatever is still unspoiled is to remain unspoiled, and to decree that all humanity, including all its technologists and scientists and leaders and other geniuses, is henceforth to concentrate on improving the places it has already marked up. Society has enough information now to begin saying something like this: we now have more access than we need, more speed and mobility than we can handle, and more people than we can survive; we do not now have all the diversity of other living things that we had or that we need or that we should give a chance to share our ride. Say that and mean it, and Maui will endure.

"What are we after?" Justice Douglas posed the question to himself at the University of Hawaii seminar. He had spoken a requiem for vanishing quiet: only in the Brooks Range of Alaska, in the American Southwest, in the Northwest—only there did stillness remain. He knew the importance of rearranging lives, government, and conscience toward the land so that serenity could survive. "It's still worth trying," he said, and asked, "What's your alternative?" What we are after? "An environment in some kind of balance, in which everything has a chance to live."

Everything. The wolf, the deer, the great goshawk, their living food, and ourselves. All came from the one source, shaped by different adversities into a stable, complex, beautiful, essential, living diversity. That source was the first cell; on Tuesday noon in the week of creation, it took it upon itself to split—a process which, beginning there, has never failed once in the building of a direct line from then to now and to each of us here and each living thing there is. From myth and from science we know about this miracle; we take it for granted—and self-inflict a monstrous deprivation. We deny ourselves a sense of wonder, of dream, of miracle.

Something happened to us on Maui that keeps the miracle from being commonplace. Thanks to Mr. Sam Pryor's concern not only about endangered places but also about endangered species, in this case a two-and-a-half-year-old gibbon he had rescued from illegal confinement in a Hong Kong petshop, we were privileged to watch Kip, the gibbon, enjoy unconfined moments in untrammeled country. Much of his day must be in a cage, for he is not likely to fit properly, unrestrained, into the Mauian ecosystem. But in the morning, Mr. Pryor joins him for cornflakes, coffee, and brachiation in a breakfast room freshly cleared of all brachiable furniture. Then Sam Pryor walks through the garden and along a bit of narrow road, Kip's arm around his neck, until they cross an old rail fence. That is the freedom signal, and Kip is off on his own, untethered, the unordered jungle growth of Maui all his. We follow.

In the Central Park menagerie and the Bronx zoo I have often watched, entranced, while the gibbons make the most of their cages, performing gymnastic feats quite beyond my poor kinesthetic powers, but beautiful nonetheless. Anyone who has thus watched gibbons knows full well that they never require support and never really touch anything. They are supported wholly, and are powered wholly, by rhythm. Nothing else. For what else could create this beauty of timing and precision and fluid motion?

Suddenly to see this miracle free, with no bars, no ceiling, no disapproval, was to learn at last what jungle growth was for, and why branches are spaced the way they are and of varying thickness and resiliency, and how those that are long enough for swinging on are just strong enough not to break, even if only pencil-thin and caught on the fly after a death-defiant twenty-foot leap through jungle-top space. So much for my teleologist's view. Kip was off into the upperstory, rappelling to walk the ground awkwardly, arms up and circling for balance, staggering for a few feet, flowing horizontally along a row of thin vertical stems by swinging in discrete arcs on alternate sides, as he rhythmed from stem to stem, glancing gently off our heads, *en passant*, if we happened to be conveniently on his route, arm-springing aloft again, fleeing precipitously to hide silent and unseen in the treetops, shortly to reappear and keep us company if we moved on. He was competent in his green world, and it returned the compliment.

When we had circled and were near the rail fence again he knew all was over. His unseen silence then became protracted, in spite of Sam Pryor's entreating calls, so Sam lay down and moaned to feign all but mortal injury. With a rush, Kip materialized out of the green of his heaven, wavered along a high branch, swung to a second tree and then another, all at the third-story level, leapt to a drooping branch, slithered the length of it, dropped recklessly to the ground and raced over it to jump on Sam's chest and embrace him. It was all a ruse—Pryor planning —but it was also a game, and Kip knew he would be free soon. I will be freer myself whenever I remember him, and be glad there are gibbons to share a planet with.

Conceding as we do that we are the world's most intelligent creatures, we ought to be bright enough to give Albert Schweitzer's reverence for life a better try. That reverence comes easier, I find, when I have taken the time to learn a little about how other creatures operate. I don't find it necessary to ask, What good is a gibbon? That is a question for other gibbons to answer. I will settle for a little envy of the way gibbons coincide with their environment and wish man success in trying to blend as well. Their senses seem all to be working beautifully. Ours aren't. Perhaps it is about time for man to try to come back to his senses, all of them, better than he does when too enamoured of his overriding technology and overbearing intellect. Where could we come to our senses better than out of doors? That is what our senses were built to cope with well, for all but this miniscule fraction of man's time on earth.

What we need is not an expanding economy, but an expanding individual. Howard Gossage told me this, hardly two months before leukemia spent a great man too soon. Maui, I think, still suggests that the individual can expand, and have no trouble understanding other living things, if he can manage to renounce some of his dependence on man-made ephemera and to spend more time with things as they were, are, and may still be.

DAVID R. BROWER
President, Friends of the Earth

Berkeley, California
May 31, 1970

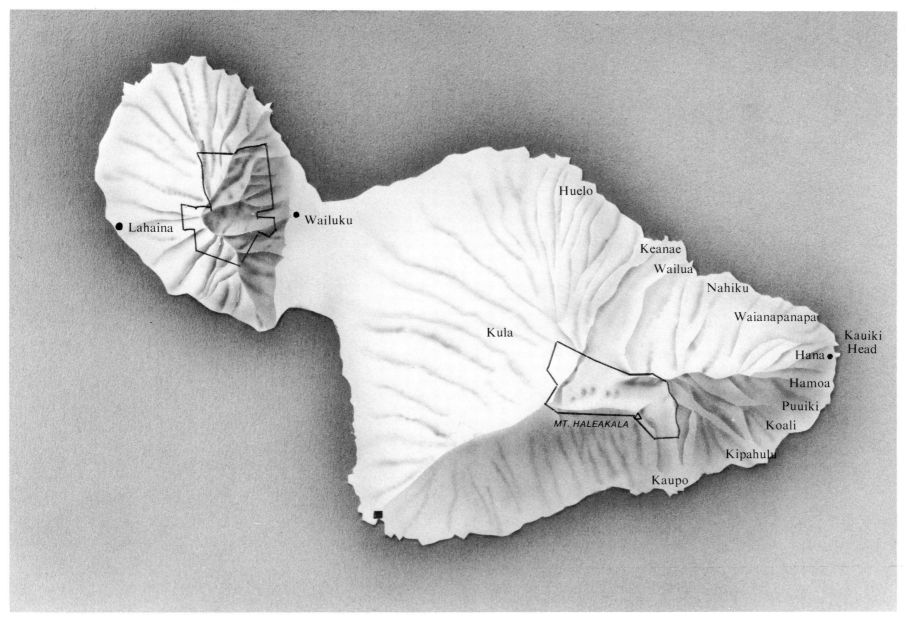

West and East Maui: scale, six miles to the inch, by James Cutter.

The grandeur and the tranquillity of Maui's Haleakala has always been an influence upon my inner spirit. Born on Maui, I am a child of its seashore, its tropical jungles, its streams and valleys. Let this book be dedicated to the human effort now needed to preserve them, that those who come after us will have the opportunity to enjoy their beauty. Nature's extravagance is resplendent on Maui. May we always want to return there.

PATSY T. MINK, *Member of Congress, Hawaii*

INTRODUCTION

Midway across the North Pacific, space, time, and life uniquely interlace a chain of islands named "Hawaiian." For two thousand miles, no continental coast exists to prop their bulging ocean. These small fragments of land appear offered to sky by water and pressed to earth by stars. Circling our world eastward, one crosses the dateline to meet them in yesterday. Circling westward, one ascends from them to tomorrow. On them, today's hours come and go at tidal tempo. Here, civilizations of Occident and Orient are merging under the tropic-softened influence of Polynesian culture.

Close to the Hawaiian's eastern reach, eyesight north and westward from Mauna Loa's vomitings, is the volcanic island of Maui—a short flight distant from Honolulu or from Hilo. This island, named after the demigod whose fish hook pulled up the ocean bed, is forty-five

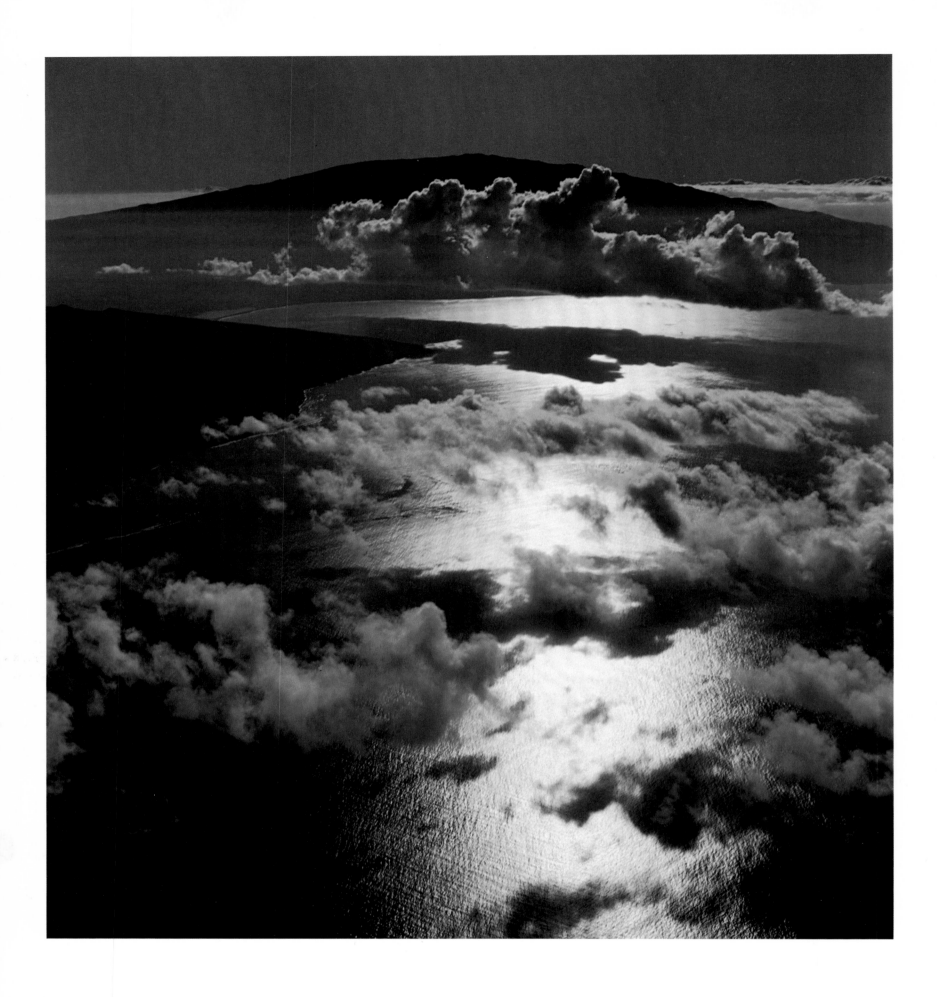

miles long and thirty miles wide as measured on a mariner's chart. Its third dimension runs from nearly two miles above to more than two miles below the surface.

Approaching through clear air, you are first aware of high slopes that curve gently downward to a flat horizon. Then line gives way to color, to the dark spongy green of jungle and the dark rippled blue of sea, separated by a white ravelling of surf—or to the lighter green of cattle ranges and pineapple fields. Flying over the high volcano, you see that in a single swoop Maui's terrain changes from moonlike desert to breadfruit trees on a leaf-lush coast.

On this coast park-bound passengers transfer from plane to automobile for the climb to Haleakala's huge, extinct, and cone-pocked crater—where colors interplay with clouds, snow descends in winter, and the twisting fury of past centuries lies petrified in flow.

Seated on some high, bleak ledge, you watch a foot trail angle down the crater rim and wind off into desert—apparently stumbling over the abrasive rocks as a man stumbles when he walks. Is it possible that beyond the rough-edged, distant ridge—hours of trudging but minutes of flight away—are rain forests, coconut palms, and naked brown children on beaches? That you will spend your afternoon in lunar settings and still drive down for supper in a country where orchids bloom, wild pigs root, and valleys thunder with a thousand waterfalls?

In early morning, you can stand on one of Maui's beaches and watch day break in either east or west, judging by pinkness of cloud—the double sunrise of Pacific islands. The constant roar of a white cascade behind you is answered by periodic roars of white-foam waves in front. Depending on which way you turn, you wade into freshwater pools or dive through a breaking sea.

Swimming out beyond the surf, you look down on waving fronds and coral-bearing reefs. Hundreds of fish surround you, weightless in the water—large and small, brilliantly hued; parrots, angels, butterflies, tunas. Some drift to deeper channels when you come too near. Some dart into crevices. You see langouste antenna in holes between rocks; and if you raise your head, porpoises may jump or a humpback whale may spout.

Exploring the coastline, now on beach, now on cliff, you soon make contact with both Maui's history and modern culture. Bush-sprouting, loose-stone foundations mark house sites of generations past. Higher walls are the ruins of religious temples, where Kane, Kanaloa, Ku, and Lono were the major gods. Men and women about them show how islands blend the races of our world. In this blending, you see Hawaii's past entering its future and recognize the value of establishing great parks.

The Hawaiian Islands will continue to ride their bulge of ocean, to appear held up by water and pressed down by stars; but Hawaiians are no longer Polynesians, and the centuries of isolated life are past. Immigration from Europe, America, and Asia has overwhelmed the native population. Primitive ways have almost disappeared. The impact of twentieth-century transportation, economics, and politics will produce results as far beyond our present vision as statehood and hotel-ridden Waikiki were beyond a Hawaiian's vision a hundred years ago.

What balance between good and evil our civilized ways will bring, we cannot now foretell; but experience shows that they destroy unprotected wilderness and wild life with appalling ruthlessness; and that, unlike man's civilizations, destroyed nature cannot be rebuilt. Once violated it is gone forever, as is the ancient beauty of Waikiki beach.

Most of Maui's natural beauty still exists; but with tourists and citizens increasing yearly by the thousands, it can be kept only through such acts of preservation as extending Haleakala National Park to include the valley of Seven Pools and a thousand waterfalls, and stretches of their ruin-monumented, spray-lashed, life-abounding coast.
CHARLES A. LINDBERGH

While much of Hawaii has become one of the most famous resorts in the world, Maui Island, developing intelligently, has remained the Hawaii spoken of in song and legend. Untarnished by clusters of highrise hotels and smog-producing freeways. Maui offers the visitor and resident a way of life unquestionably unique in the world.

Maui possesses open space, long-range planning opportunities, historical traditions, and scenic resources on such a grand scale that many thousands of additional tourists and residents can be welcomed without sacrificing her aloha spirit or her unequalled warmth, charm, and native beauty. The orderly planning of Maui Island's growth and the preservation of her scenic resources in a greatly expanded national park, combined with increased recreational opportunities in larger state and county parks, offer positive ways to preserve the treasures of Maui for our visitors and our citizens today and for generations yet to come.

ELMER F. CRAVALHO, *Mayor, County of Maui*

Hydrogen bomb aurora, red night sky, Haleakala

Prologue

The constellation the Greeks called Orion was called Na Kao by the early Hawaiians. The Hawaiians, who watched Na Kao march across the zenith every winter night, saw him as a giant warrior. They saw darts on his belt, darts that split the clouds over island peaks and brought down the sacred rains. He held a favored place in the Hawaiian heaven, along with Naholoholo, the western evening star.

Na Kao was still below the horizon an hour before

THE LAST HAWAIIAN PLACE

midnight in July 1962, as a small group of warmly clothed men, 10,000 feet high on Maui's Mount Haleakala, watched Naholoholo assume his place in the sky and blend with the wide sweep of the Milky Way. Occasionally a shooting star darted toward the distant horizon. The night was clear and cloudless. A chilling breeze rustled the plants that grew between the jumbled basalt blocks scattered across the summit.

The men who stood on the summit, and their colleagues, had built what seemed a moon station on the volcanic mountain. The cold black lava of the southwest rift zone now supported Air Force trailers bristling with electronic gear and radar screens. Occasionally, from the direction of the trailers, a shaft of light pierced the darkness, and momentarily revealed a silhouetted figure darting into the doorway of the instrument-laden Atomic Energy Commission van.

A shortwave radio, lying between the legs of a photographer's tripod, fed back static gathered from the air between Maui and Johnson Island, 800 miles distant in the South Pacific. The noise was interrupted at intervals by an unemotional voice giving the countdown to zero. It was a monotonous countdown, begun abortively five times during the week. Tonight it would be completed. The Thor rocket was off its pad on Johnson Island and rising rapidly into the night.

The usually familiar stars of the Milky Way seemed unreal tonight as scientists, armed guards, and photographers peered intently toward the southwest. The countdown continued for several minutes. The sky seemed to move and then wait, as the unknown voice rose higher in pitch and began to speak in seconds. The photographer opened his camera shutters and waited for zero.

There was no sound. In the briefest of instants, the world was gone. There was no color and no shape, all was empty and white. There was nothing to see or feel. The sky, sea, and earth were wiped out in a white glare.

Just as suddenly, there was darkness again. But now stars were gone. The night closed in quickly and pushed against the startled human figures huddled on the mountain. A bright green star appeared where none had existed before and with horrible swiftness, grew monstrously into an exploding ball of fire—800 miles away and 240 miles above the earth's surface, yet at arm's length. No one dared reach out.

The silent flame changed in seconds from green to bloody red, then irresistibly spread its bright stain across space, polluting the heavens, the afterbirth of a hydrogen bomb.

The stars came out again. The Milky Way glowed anew against the sky. Doors opened and stayed ajar, the familiar yellow light casting reassuring shadows across the lunar landscape, though high-energy electrons in the ionosphere continued to glow in long arcs across the sky, dramatically revealing the earth's magnetic field between north and south poles. Rainbow curtains of an artificially induced aurora borealis shimmered in the north in the eternity before the heavens stopped bleeding.

Then Na Kao, the warrior constellation, rose and joined Naholoholo in the sky. The technicians packed up and departed, and the heavens seemed almost the same.

The small installation remained on Haleakala's summit. Called "Science City" by the people of Maui, it continues to investigate, with telescope and camera, the wilderness of space. Entrance to its laboratories is restricted. Signs are posted reminding visitors to stay on the pavement so that rising dust will not obscure the heavens. At night, travelers on Haleakala's high road are asked to dim their headlights so that the faintest glimmerings from outer galaxies will be recorded.

But below the telescope is another wilderness. A desert of cinder slopes in one direction, a deep jungle in the other, it minimizes Science City just as overwhelmingly as the universal wilderness minimizes our planet. Miles away, where this smaller wilderness meets the wilderness of the sea, lower down where the air is warmer and the nights more fragrant, lives a Hawaiian lady named Annie Smith, in a comfortable house with clean white interior and woven mats on the floor. Annie Smith remembers the sugar-plantation days on her part of the coast. And several miles away, by the electric light he introduced to this coast, an old Chinese storekeeper and inventor, Nick Soon, a man who remembers when the Hawaiians in his district lived in grass houses, assorts his latest color slides.

This book is about the memories, about the history and possible future, of these people and their older world. It is written from an unease concerning the new world of Science City and the green star that grew so monstrously above it, written with the conviction that the new world must find a place for the old.

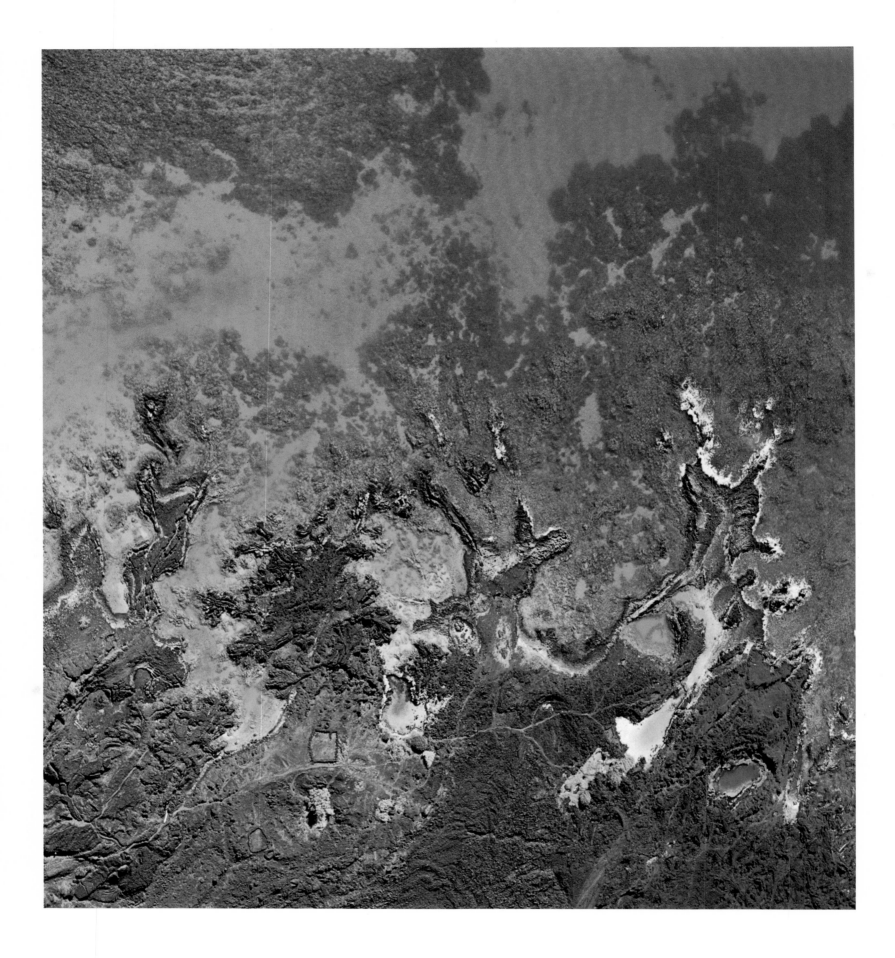

1. Origins

THE HIGH SUMMIT crater of Haleakala was still venting molten lava when the ancestors of the Hawaiians began moving eastward in their long migration across the Pacific. The ancestors settled in the Samoan islands about 1500 B.C., then sailed farther eastward to the Marquesas, where they paused and prospered. Sometime between 200 and 400 years before Christ, they moved again, this time dispersing to Easter Island, Tahiti, and Hawaii.

The voyagers had no written language, and traditions were passed on orally, through chants. In this old but sure way, stories of the homeland were carried across the seas and generations to new children born in lands unknown to their grandparents. And so it was that as the first Hawaiians stepped ashore after the long, arduous voyage from the Marquesas, the new land had a familiar look. The volcanic islands they saw looked exactly as their Samoan home, Savaii, had been described to them. They named the biggest island Savaii, or Hawaii. Then they crossed the channel from Hawaii and landed on the island to the north, pulling their waterlogged canoes ashore at a spot they named Samoa, or Hamoa. This second island, with its new Samoa, was named Maui after the Polynesian demigod who had safely escorted the travelers across the pathless seas.

Stories of the demigod Maui are recounted in exotic languages to the inhabitants of primitive villages scattered across some thirteen million square miles of sea and land, from the atolls of Micronesia to the lonely islands of Hawaii, many weeks' sail north from Tahiti and the Marquesas. *"Ko Maui tinihanga koe,"* "You Maui of a thousand tricks, you," is the Maori version of a maternal reprimand common to a thousand Pacific islands. Royalty of almost every Pacific land claims Maui as an ancestor. In the Hawaiian Islands, King Kalakaua and Queen Liliuokalani noted him in their genealogies.

Maui was neither man nor god. He deserted the gods of the underworld to join man, but proved a misfit on earth, warped by the attempted abortion that had denied him a full nine-months' shelter in his mother's womb.

Originally, when he lived beneath the earth, Maui had eight heads. He tore seven of them off, one by one, in order to climb through a small hole that led to the surface. The sunlight was pleasant, and Maui decided to live above ground. Now all men who live on the surface of the Earth have only one head.

Maui was not satisfied with the first man created. First Man could not move. His arms and legs were jointless and his limbs were webbed. Maui took First Man and broke him at the ankles, knees, and hips to create joints. He tore the limbs loose from their webs of skin so that man could move about. And it was Maui, many islanders claim, who lifted the heavy skies high enough that man could walk upright instead of crawling on all fours.

Maui starved his blind grandmother to get her jawbone as a magical weapon. Then he cut off his own ear for bait, and using the jawbone as a fishhook, pulled up many sizes and varieties of fish from the ocean. His catch became Pacific islands.

According to the *Kumulipo*, a Hawaiian creation chant that ties Maui's adventures together in an epic series, Maui also used his mother's pet mudhen as bait. The pet's wing was broken off in Maui's struggle to wrest the bird from his mother, and when he fished with the imperfect bait, he caught a broken-up land—the Hawaiian Islands.

After fishing up the Hawaiian Islands, Maui tried to unite them into a single unbroken group, an ambitious undertaking that required him to meet One Tooth, a supernatural being who lived beneath the sea near the entrance to Pearl Harbor. One Tooth was responsible for holding the newly caught islands and keeping them from drifting too close together or too far apart. In order to make a single continent of Hawaii, Maui had to persuade this demon to let go. One Tooth, unfortunately, like all beings of a higher order, disliked Maui. He was offended by the slightest suggestion that he change his way of doing things, and denied Maui's request. Rebuffed, Maui went to a cave near Nanakuli Beach on Oahu and consulted his mother, who advised him to go far offshore before returning to meet One Tooth again. Far from land he would find something to help him, she told him.

When he had sailed so far out that the Waianae mountains were hazy on the horizon, Maui found a bailing calabash floating on the waves and recognized it immediately as the help his mother had promised. He placed the calabash in a safe place and he and his brothers, who had accompanied him on his expedition, paddled steadily back toward Pearl Harbor. As they drew near, the cala-

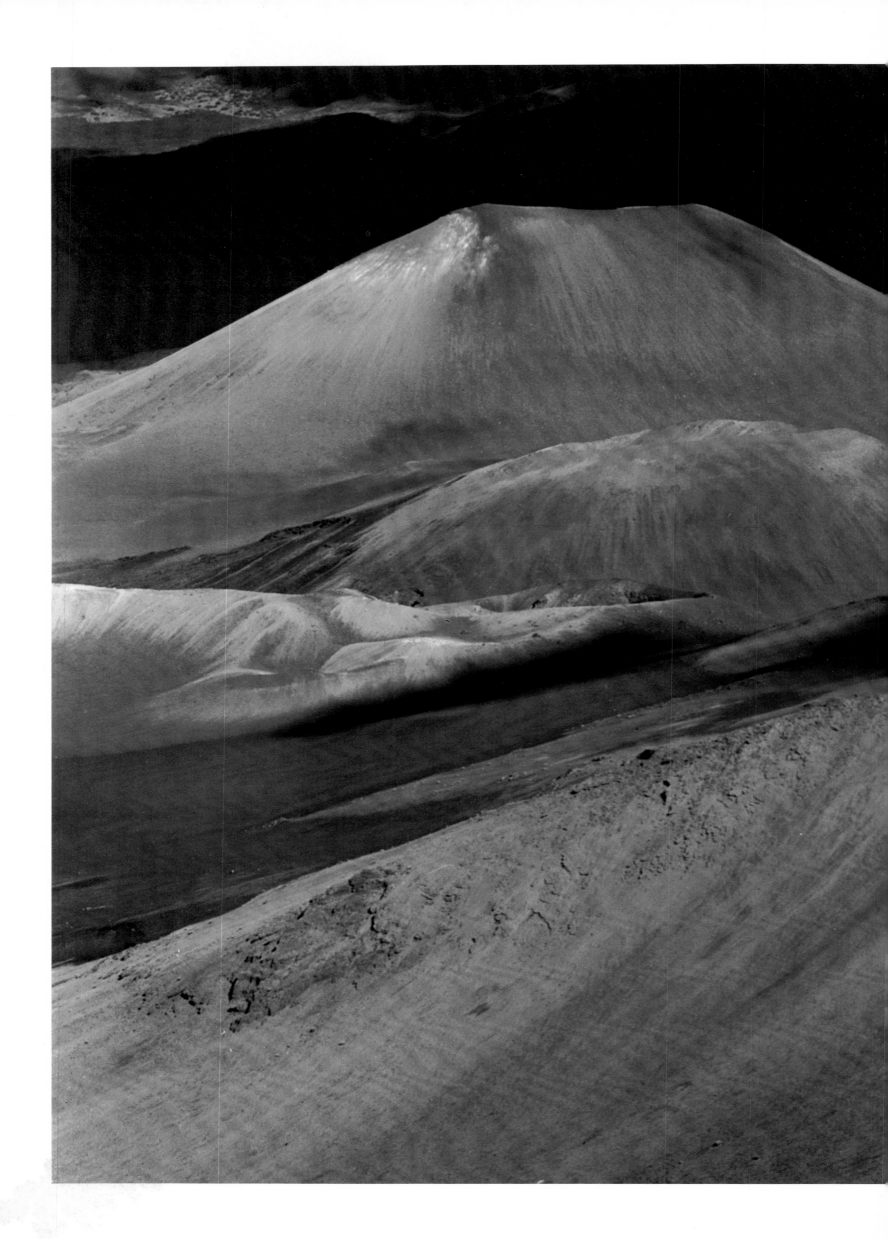

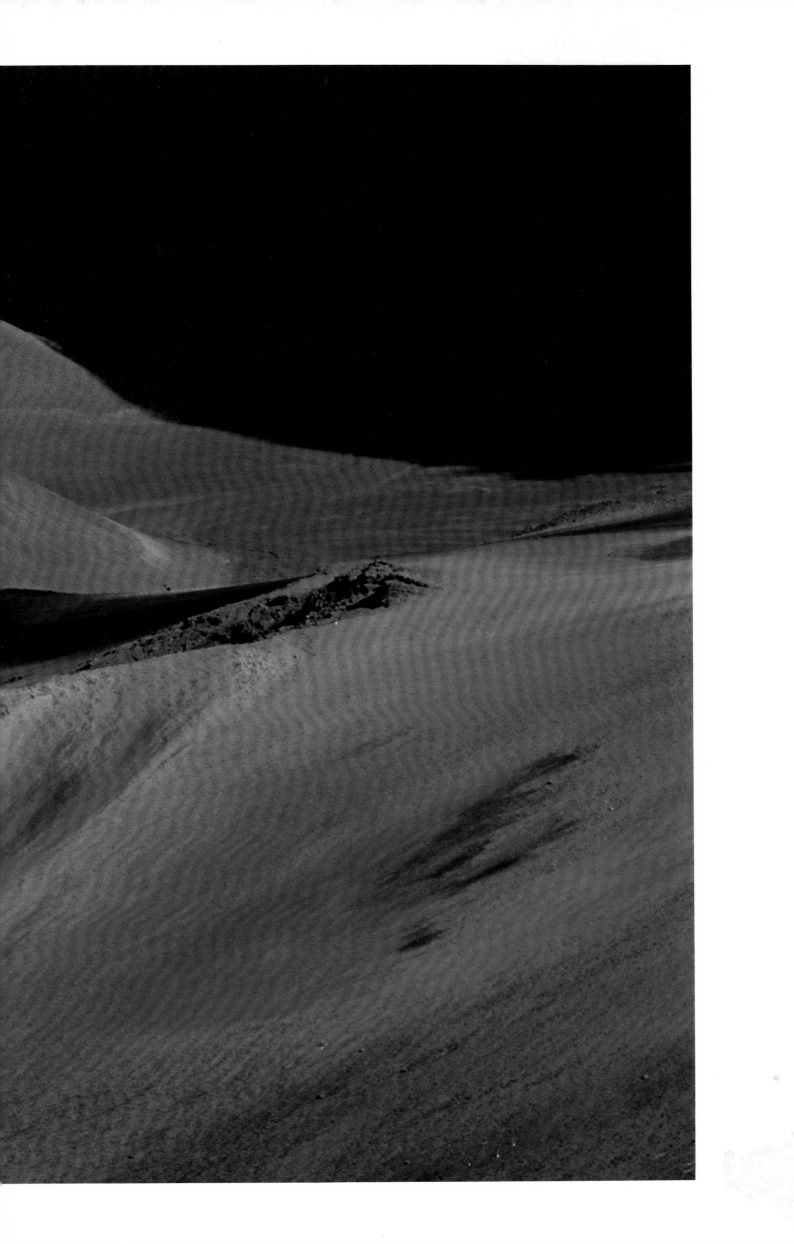

bash became a beautiful young mermaid, Hina, the Moon Lady. Before Maui could cast anchor, however, the brown mermaid disappeared, leaving only the calabash on the bottom of the canoe. Maui angrily threw it overboard and prepared to meet old One Tooth on his own.

Maui's plan was to fish for One Tooth, hook him, and force him to release the islands. Maui first caught several sharks for practice, then took out his magic jawbone and tossed his line in the water. The Moon Lady, who was not annoyed at having been tossed overboard, was waiting below, and pulled the hook under without revealing herself above the waves. She carried it deep into the sea until she came to One Tooth. She approached him seductively, and One Tooth was forced to smile. He revealed his famous single tooth. Hina quickly tossed the hook down his throat when his mouth opened, then threw two loops of sennit around the lone tooth. Maui, floating anxiously in the canoe above, felt the strike. He secured the line and exhorted his brothers to paddle with all their strength. He warned them not to look back under any circumstances. The brothers paddled steadily to the northwest, but grew restless as Maui urged them on, and soon could no longer restrain their curiosity. They glanced back and exclaimed at what they saw. A string of islands—Hawaii, Maui, Molokai, Oahu, and Kauai—were caught on Maui's line and splashing along behind.

The brothers shouted, "Look at what you've caught!" The charm was broken, and the carefully placed hook slipped from One Tooth's mouth. The islands stopped in their forward movement, scattered and slipped. They churned in the water, and Kauai and Niihau spun about together near the canoe. The line snapped and hurled the others farther away toward Tahiti. But One Tooth recovered his senses in time and was able to hold Hawaii Island in place near a hot part of the ocean floor. He caught Oahu as it began to float away and, before tending to his aching mouth, stopped Molokai from jamming into the island bearing Maui's name. Maui was gone by the time One Tooth got his fish again under control, spread out much as they had been when Maui's line snapped. Not daring to take further chances, One Tooth tied them all to the ocean floor where he found them—in the places where they are today.

Maui once lived at Makaliua on West Maui. It was from here that he brought off his greatest Hawaiian exploit.

The days were short on Maui Island. The gathering of bark and pounding of tapa required all day, and there was insufficient time remaining after pounding the wet tapa for it to dry before the sun dipped below the mountain rim. No time remained for the people to cook their food before dark and bring in the fishing nets they had laid out before dawn.

Maui resolved to snare the sun and halt its swift flight across the sky. He wove a cord from his sister's pubic hair, twisted it into throw lengths, and with these thrown over his shoulder, climbed to the summit of Haleakala, House of the Sun, and there awaited the light above the eastern rim. When the Sun God stood full against the eastern sky, Maui lassoed him between the legs, a fighting technique that later Polynesian warriors would practice on their enemies. Maui beat the Sun God with the magic jawbone, permanently crippling him. The maimed sun now moves slowly across the sky, and gives the people time to dry their tapa, bring in the nets, carefully extract the small fish caught in the mesh, and cook before dark.

The adventure that brought about Maui's death was more inspired than any that he succeeded in. It began innocently enough: For a joke Maui transformed his sister's husband into a dog. The villagers made him an outcast for this, and he was forced to live with his father beneath the earth. It was there that he first heard of his powerful ancestress, Great Hina of the underworld, whose character was as warped as his own. She was one of the first women the great god Tane had created when he was experimenting with people. Hina was beautiful, and was such an accomplishment that Tane did not reveal that he was her father, and took her as his wife. When Hina learned the truth she became a cruel destroyer of men. Maui vowed now to vanquish her.

Since Maui was at this time an outcast, the only warriors he could find to accompany him were pretty birds. As Maui approached Hina, who was sleeping on her back, the birds were terrified. Maui told them not to be afraid. They would shortly see something funny, he assured them, and he warned them not to wake Hina with their laughter. To kill the goddess, and to become immortal himself, Maui intended to crawl into her body and out her mouth.

The awed warrior birds fluttered quietly overhead, watching as Maui crawled between Great Hina's thighs. Maui's head disappeared, then his broad shoulders and chest. Hina did not stir. Finally only his legs stuck out, a funny sight. A rippling titter ran among the birds. The goddess awoke, saw what was happening, and, squeezing her legs together, crushed Maui.

Maui's flesh had proven mortal, but his cosmic mischievousness did not. His deeds have lived and are remembered throughout the Pacific.

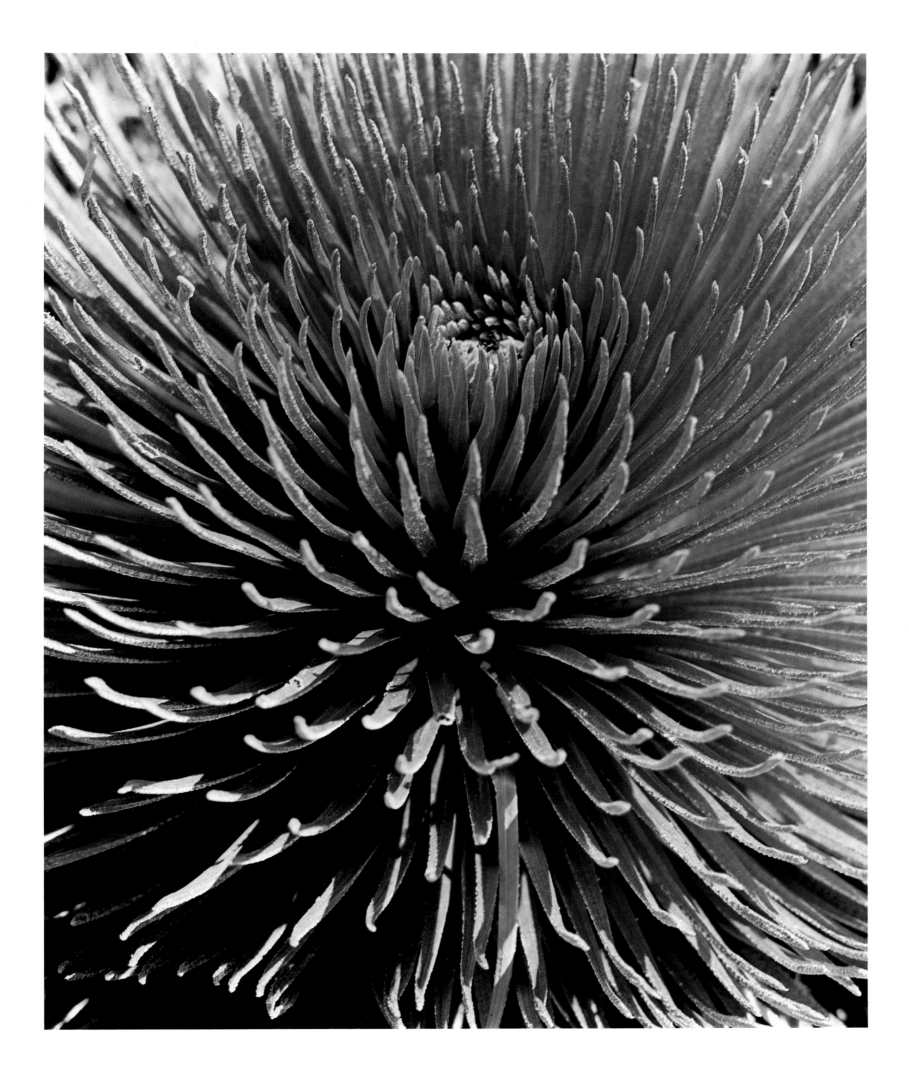

2. Hana

THE COAST of East Maui, from the first Polynesian landing place, the dry peninsula at Kaupo,
through Kipahulu to the lush taro patches of
Keanae is *aina alii*, the royal land of Hana. The inhabitants
of Hana could assume the prerogatives of royalty, it is
said, simply by being born in the place. Many of Hana's
commoners ignored the *kapus* of chiefs traveling from
other districts, and in general lived a good life, with a
measure of freedom not found elsewhere in the islands.

Hana was rich country. The common people easily
satisfied the demands of local chiefs for taro, sweet potatoes, bananas, sugar cane, and wild fruit. Fish ponds along
the shore were prolific and the deep waters beyond provided well for Hawaiians skillful with surround nets and
outrigger canoes. According to the old chants recorded by
Hawaiian historian Samuel Kamakau, Hana was famous
for "the surf at Puhele, the fresh-water bathing pool of
Kumaka, the diving at Waiohinu, the flying spray of
Kama, the changing color of the fronds of the ama'u fern,
the yellow-leafed awa of Lanakila, the delicious poi of
Kuakani, the fat opihi shellfish of Kawaipapa, the fat soft
uhu fish of Haneo'o, and the juicy pork and tender dog
meat dear to the memory of chiefs of that land."

Hana is the lanai of Mount Haleakala. Its gently sloping land reposes like the green entrance of an old plantation house. Hana faces the sunrise and enjoys fresh sea and
land winds. There are two sea winds; one, called *Kohala-
pehu*, brings rain and is followed by a dry calm, the other,
Kohala-pele, drives away the clouds from Alenuihaha Channel, clearing the view to Hawaii Island. The land breeze,
Lau'awa, blows gently down the open slopes of Haleakala
into Hana Bay, bringing with it the fragrance of *hala*.

Weather was a great fact for the people of Hana. They
were residents of an island. Their horizons were circum-
scribed, their geography limited in its possibilities, their
seasons hard to distinguish. What variety they had was
meteorological. They lived under the sky and were sensi-
tive to its changes. They had a name for every mood of
the weather.

Hana's most famous rain is called the *apuakea*, and it
falls after sunrise, rattling the dry hala leaves as the shower
sweeps over the shore. The wet months of the year are
called *ho'oilo*—whimsical months, when the rain showers

heavily on Kaeleku, perhaps, and bypasses Hamoa with
hardly a sprinkle. In the late afternoons of ho'oilo, squalls
move in from the gray ocean, blow across taro fields, and,
leaving the taro leaves wet and washed, continue on to
upland rain forests.

It was in Hana that the most momentous love affair in
Maui's history took place.

Chief Kiha-a-Piilani, the son of the ruling chief of
Maui, was one of the lovers. Kiha had learned to surf on
the long waves of Waikiki, and the smaller waves of Hana
left much to be desired. The best surf near Hana was at
Keanini along the west corner of Hana Bay, a favorite
surfing place of Chiefess Kumaka, a daughter of the chief
of Hana, who was betrothed to Kiha's brother. Kiha
joined Kumaka at the beach one day, and Kumaka, standing upright on her heavy *olo* board of *wiliwili* wood, taught
him the trick of mastering the short surf at Keanini. On
one occasion when the waves ran long, the two were
carried to the beach together and, exhilarated by the ride,
they lay together on the beach and made love. Kumaka's
desire for Kiha's brother Lono, the man her father intended she marry, quickly faded.

Kumaka returned to Keanini again and again afterward,
but Kiha failed to appear. She searched for him and found
him at his family home. Kiha, learning that she was
pregnant, left and went to live with her.

When the news reached Kumaka's father, he was in-
furiated. He had placed a kapu upon her—no one but
Lono could marry her. Kumaka had broken the kapu and
rejected the planned union. Her father disowned her, be-
lieving the marriage to be part of a conspiracy by Kiha to
dispose of his brother Lono, who was, as royal brothers
often were, a political rival. When Kumaka asked for a
division of the Hana lands upon the birth of a son, her
father refused, saying, "I shall not take Kiha's part. I shall
remain loyal to his older brother till these bones perish.
Your husband does not want farm lands for the two of
you, but is seeking means to rebel against the kingdom.
The lands of Honoma'ele and Ka'eleku he requests supply
the *ohia* wood and *ie ie* vines for the ladders of the fortress
Ka'uiki. Kawaipapa supplies the stones that are used in
battle. The Wananalua lands hold the fortress and the

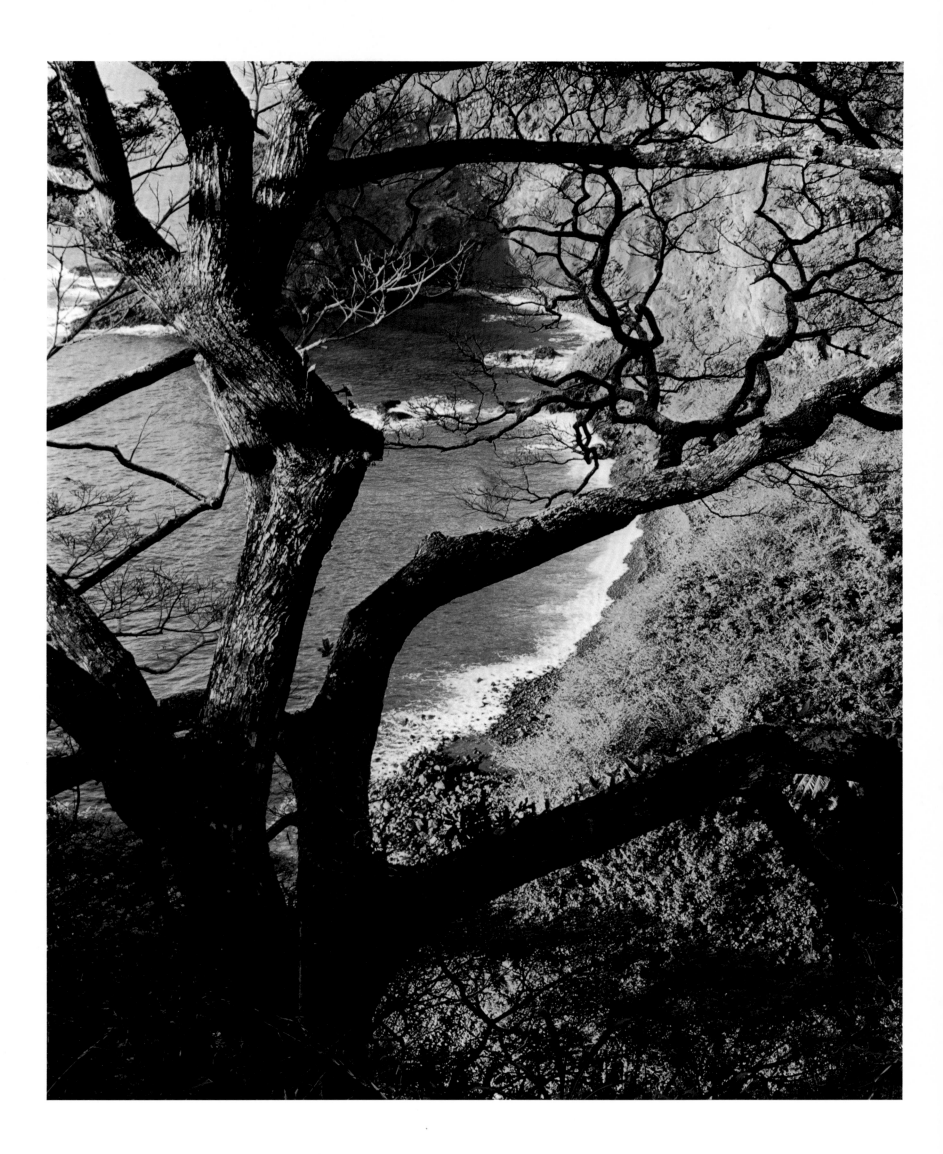

places below it. I shall not take your husband's side." With this, he dismissed Kumaka, and took her son to rear as his own.

Chief Kiha's brother-in-law was Umi-a-Liloa, the young, ambitious chief of northern Hawaii Island, who saw in the family quarrel an opportunity to extend his influence across the channel. When Umi's brothers-in-law went to war against each other, Umi took sides with the younger brother. He vowed to avenge the wrongs committed against Kiha and Kumaka. Lono, in his turn, was supported by a powerful Maui chief. Kumaka, then, became Hawaii's Helen—a stolen woman who set armies at odds. When the two alliances met, the confrontation was an epic one, Hawaii's Trojan War.

Umi-a-Liloa planned a massive assault on Maui across thirty-five miles of rough channel waters to the shores of Hana. His warriors and serfs spent an entire year con-

Umi's great fleet was repulsed in its first assault on the Maui shore. His warriors were forced to retreat from landings at Ka'uiki fortress and the beaches at Hamoa and Punahoa by the spears and slingstones of Lono's men. The defeated Hawaiians fled to the open sea in disorder. The fleet lay off Maui that night, the invaders nursing their wounds and preparing for morning. At dawn, Umi's men renewed their assault. His canoes crowded ashore at every possible landing place, but the defense was invincible. Heavy *ala* stones swamped canoes loaded with warriors before they reached shore. Smooth flat pebbles from the beach at Waianapanapa smashed into the unprotected heads of men carrying canoes ashore at Hana. Some canoes were splintered by huge boulders, others were seized, and the rest put in disorder by the stone-slinging young Maui defenders.

When Umi arrived in the bloody waters off Hana with a later wave of men, he realized that he could not conquer

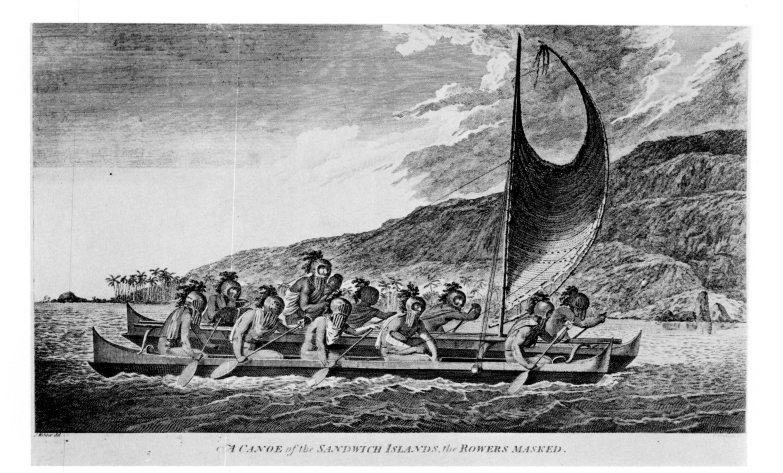

A CANOE of the SANDWICH ISLANDS, the ROWERS MASKED.

structing double war canoes, carving spears, and chipping war clubs of *kauila* wood. When the expedition began, Umi's great fleet of canoes, in numbers never before seen in Hawaii, filled Alenuihaha Channel from shore to shore, the first canoes reaching Hana before the last pushed off from Hawaii. It was 1300 A.D., and the first invasion of another island in Hawaiian history.

Maui from the sea. Directed by his ally Kiha, he sailed to a small landing many miles northwest of Hana, where an overland attack could be mounted. At the Wailua-iki landing the canoes were dismantled as fast as they touched bottom on the tiny black beach and were set upright against the sea cliff so that all could be brought ashore.

The overland fighting began on the cliffs above and

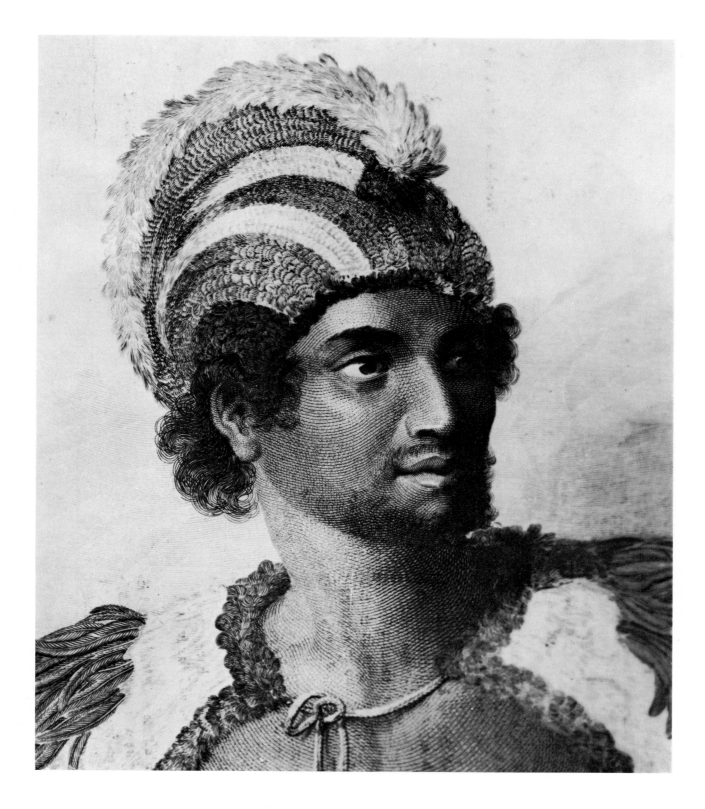

might see in advance whether nobility was approaching. The straightness of the Highway also helped the chiefs guard against ambush.

The trail began on the wide, sloping tongue of lava that protrudes into the sea at Kaupo. Here the early Maui people lived in a large village settlement, the most densely populated community on East Maui. In its first sixteen miles, the Highway wound in and out of the numerous green gulches that lie between Kaupo and Hana. Traveling this stretch of the trail was an adventure. When seas were smooth, a piece of tapa in payment might encourage a fisherman to ferry a heavily burdened traveler around the next point in his canoe, but otherwise the traveler had to rely on his ingenuity. When mountain cloudbursts swelled the streams, he had to swing himself across the flood-waters on ropes made of the vines that hung from nearby *kukui* trees. At Wailua Valley the trail climbed steeply up high cliffs, and natives would shorten their trip by swimming around the rocky headlands—but only when the presence of porpoises made likely the absence of sharks.

Going down the cliffs was considerably easier. A group of travelers would sit one behind the other on a sled of breadfruit branches or *ti* plants, and with a brisk kick backward, descend quickly in a dusty slide to the bottom.

The Highway was of considerable value to the chiefs, whose runners sped rapidly between different districts with messages of war or demands on the commoners for pigs and poi. Runners carried a known possession of the king so that they would be received with full confidence and allowed to pass on the trail in safety. The training of a *kukini*, or runner, involved severe hardship, but the prestige was almost that of a battle hero. The runner practiced constantly to maintain speed over long distances. He ate no heavy food—only cooked flesh of fowl, roasted taro, and breadfruit.

Maui's fastest kukini was Keliimalolo. The story is that upon landing on Hawaii one time, he jumped into the surf before the canoes were beached and quickly ran twenty miles, returning to the beach before his companions had finished washing seawater from the canoes and dragging them ashore. When they doubted his claim, he verified it by describing a joint of sugar cane he had left at his most distant point, and then leading them to it.

Luna'auhau, tax collectors for the chiefs, also ran the trail, carrying intricately carved idols that glistened with coconut oil and made the messengers' role more impressive. The commoner was careful when he encountered the idol, for if he disrespectfully forced the collector to pass on the ocean side of the trail, his life would be in jeopardy.

After the dedication ceremonies for important heiaus the trail was alive from one end of the island to the other. The dedications involved human sacrifice, and after sacrifice it was necessary that the whole island, including the Highway, be purified. On the day of purification, called *Kaloakukolu*, the entire length of the Highway was cleared of weeds and displaced rocks were restored, with each family that lived along the trail doing its share of work in a festival spirit. At the boundary of every *ahupuaa*, or land parcel, a stone altar was erected and topped by a carved image of kukui wood, and on the altar was placed an offering of hard poi.

After work on the trail was finished and everyone retired to his village, a priest appeared, his body smeared with red clay. He entoned a chant at each altar, daubing the wooden image with red clay. Then he declared the Highway purified and open to travelers.

The Kiha-a-Piilani Highway, in peaceful times an avenue of commerce, was in violent times an avenue of war. Soon after the Highway's completion, armies from up and down Maui's coast were moving along it toward Ka'uiki Fortress in an attempt to reclaim it from the forces of Hawaii Island.

For decades Ka'uiki was a hated symbol of Hawaii's sovereignty over Maui. After Umi-a-Liloa, a succession of Hawaii chiefs held it. The fortress resisted repeated attempts of Maui warriors to scale its steep cinder slopes and overrun its summit refuge. It was intolerable to King Kahekili of Maui that Hawaii maintain this foothold on his island. He summoned loyal warriors from Wailuku to Lahaina to challenge Ka'uiki, and marched overland on the Kiha-a-Piilani Highway from Ko'olau and Kaupo, torturing enemy scouts encountered along the trail. His forces approached Hana from north and south and the enemy withdrew to Ka'uiki.

For twelve months Kahekili's men laid siege to the well-provisioned stronghold. They were costly months for Maui, and the slingstones of Ka'uiki's defenders took a great toll. The fortress was clearly impregnable to direct attack. King Kahikili wondered if there was another way, and when he heard of an old Hana man who claimed that Ka'uiki could be taken without a struggle, he commanded that the man be found and brought before him.

"Yes, it is true," the old man said. "It can be taken without a scratch, or any weariness from carrying spear or club, or from being burdened with a load of slingstones." Kahekili listened as the old man explained that Ka'uiki could be taken by simply cutting it off from its water supply. The defenders got their water, he said, from springs in the black pahoehoe lava flows that encircle Hana Bay.

Kahekili immediately ordered the springs at Punahoa, Waika-akihi, Keanini, and the ponds from Kawaipapa to Honokalani across the bay placed under continuous guard by warriors armed with spears and stone weapons.

The defenders of Ka'uiki waited until darkness, then sent out their strongest swimmers, with water gourds tied tightly around their waists. The swimmers swam quietly across the black bay to Keanini, barely breaking the surface or leaving the faintest wake. They let the gentle waves and slight breeze carry them the last yards to shore. For the final minute they remained under water, following a course among submerged rocks, until each swimmer came to his spring at the water's edge, reached above the surface to dip the cool water, and found the Maui spears waiting for him.

The defenders of Ka'uiki were killed at every spring they approached. They were denied access to their water, and in a day the situation atop Ka'uiki became desperate. Canoes were lowered from the heights in a frantic effort to escape, but most were splintered by high surf against the rocky cliffs. Those warriors who remained were slaughtered, and Ka'uiki was returned to the rule of Maui chiefs.

3. Kamehameha

IN THE TOWN of Wailuku, on the broad central plain of Maui, Chief Kahekili, ruler of Maui, held court. Kahekili came closer than any chief of his time to conquering all the islands. Chants tell of his many victories and eventual defeat in battle. They also tell of his several wives, one of them the most brilliant woman in the land, Queen Namahana. Kahekili ruled firmly, like all ruling chiefs, through an elaborate system of kapus. Women were forbidden to eat with men. People of lower rank seeking an audience with the chief were required to prostrate themselves, and when the chief's party was traveling about the country a herald ran ahead, warning the people to remove their upper garments and prostrate themselves on pain of death. As was true elsewhere in Hawaii, the commoners were serfs, and Kahekili's kingdom was a feudal one. A prescribed portion of the commoners' taro, of their pigs, and of the fish they snared was collected by the chief who ruled their *ahupuaa*—their land parcel. The commoners lived at their chief's pleasure, raising children for his army, and joining him in battle.

Into Kahekili's illustrious court, frequented by the most talented artists and finest dancers in the land, came Kekuiapo-iwa, the young wife of Keoua, who was a half-brother of the Chief of Hawaii. Four months previously Kekuiapo-iwa had undergone the important ceremony of *hoomai keiki*, "sowing a baby," yet her long hair still flowed loosely in the breeze, revealing that she was not yet *hapai*—with child. Before the young woman's arrival, Chief Kahekili had granted his wife's desire to hold her own court, and while the Queen entertained her own royal visitors at Waiehu, Kahekili introduced Kakuiapo-iwa to his court, and fell in love with her.

When Kekuiapo-iwa returned from her short visit to Maui, she was found to be pregnant, and the rumor spread quickly that the father was Chief Kahekili. Her husband Keoua ignored the gossip, but when his wife developed a yearning to eat the eyeball of a man-eating shark, aging Chief Alapa'i of Hawaii became concerned, and asked the court priests to explain her strange craving.

Chief Alapa'i recalled the rumors that the expected baby's father was his rival, Chief Kahekili, a man who coveted sovereignty over Hawaii Island, and when the priests confirmed that Kekuiapo-iwa's baby would become a killer of chiefs, Alapa'i made secret plans to destroy the infant after its birth.

Kekuiapo-iwa suffered pains of childbirth on a guesthouse lanai where she had taken shelter from a heavy tropical rain. She went inside and lay down to brace her feet against the wall for the final labor pains. Alapa'i's guards arrived shortly afterward with orders to kill the baby on it's birth, but they fell asleep, bundled as they were against the chilly weather. They were unaware that Nae-ole, a loyal follower of Kehuiapo-iwa, was standing quietly by, waiting for the baby's first cry. Hearing the cry, Nae-ole entered the house, covered the child in soft tapa laid out to receive it and carried the baby into the thunder and lightning. As he stepped outside, the sky was lit by the bright passage of a comet, and thunder sounded. Both were symbols that traditionally announced the arrival of a chief.

The child born that evening was Kamehameha, the great warrior who would conquer all the islands and become the first ruler of a united kingdom. Hidden on his birth night in a basket of *olona* fiber, Kamehameha was carried over high mountain trails deep into Waipio Valley, where Nae-ole and his wife, with a newborn child of her own, raised the new chief as a foster son.

Twenty-five years later, as a warrior in an invading army, Kamehameha returned to Maui, the island of his conception. On the gently sloping sweet-potato patches of Hamoa he took part in his first battle and fought with unusual bravery against the forces of Maui chief Kahekili —his father. He saved the life of his instructor in warfare when the tutor's feet became entangled in potato vines. While the tutor freed himself, Kamehameha held off attacking Maui warriors by grabbing them between the legs and jerking them off their feet.

The Maui men gave their skillful enemy the name *Pai'ea*, the hard-shelled crab. By all early accounts, even as a young man he was fearless and ambitious, a born leader and a favorite of Kalani'opu'u, the ruling chief of Hawaii Island.

On this first campaign, as Kamehameha rested in Hana between battles, he saw a young girl at play in the fields.

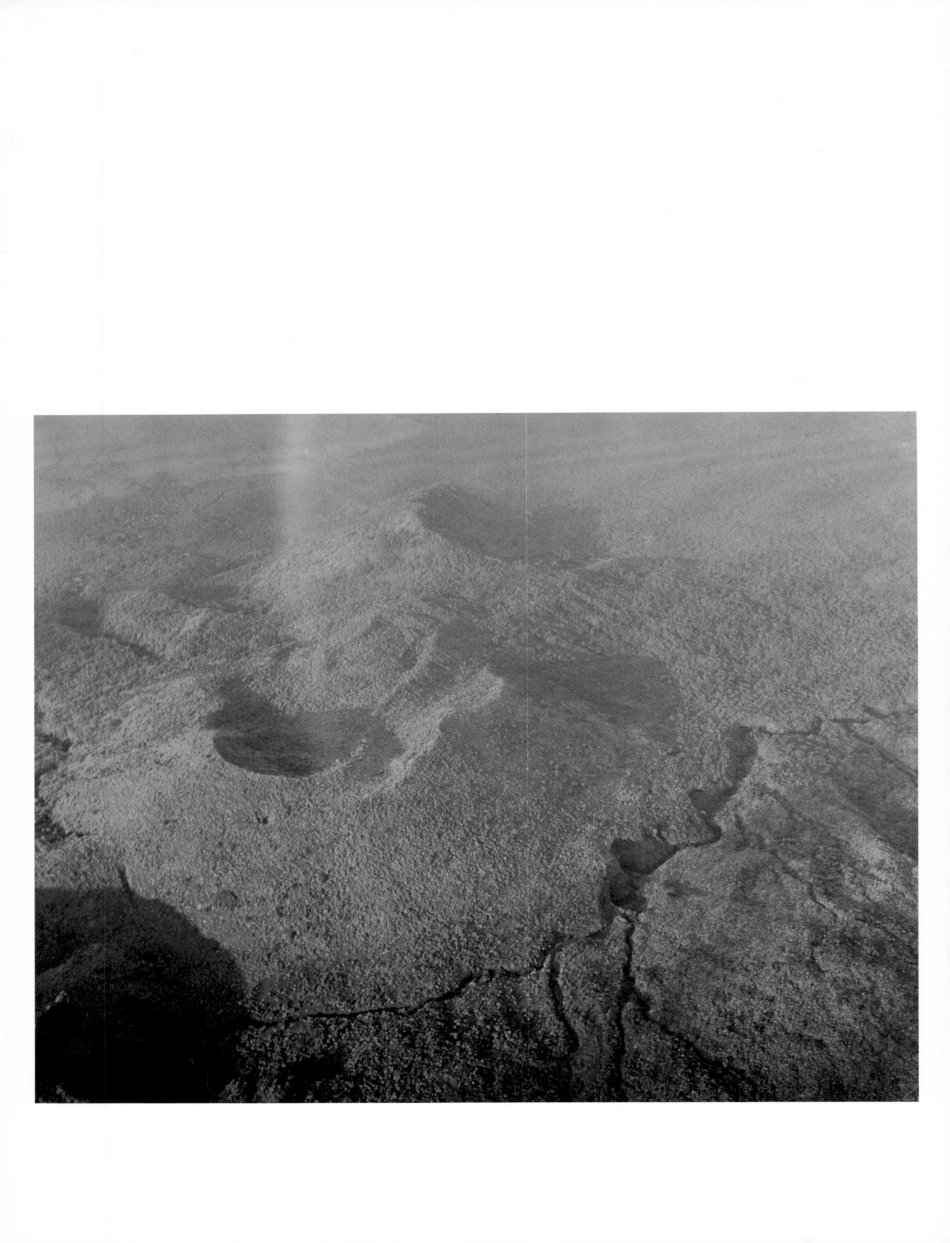

She was Ka-ahumanu, a native of Hana, born in a cave at the base of Ka'uiki Head. Though just eleven, she was beautiful, and Kamehameha decided that one day she would be his wife. Shortly after the young warrior returned to Hawaii, the girl's mother, weary of the constant warfare at Hana, fled with her family to the Big Island, and there, two years after he had first seen Ka-ahumanu, Kamehameha married her.

Hawaiian historian Samuel Kamakau, drawing on chants from Kamehameha's day, later described Ka-ahumanu as "a handsome woman, six feet tall, straight and well formed, without blemish, and comely. Her arms were like the inside of a banana stalk, her fingers tapering, her palms pliable like kukunene grass, graceful in repose, her cheeks long in shape and pink as the bud of a banana stem; her eyes like those of a dove or the moho bird; her nose narrow and straight, in admirable proportion to her cheeks; her arched eyebrows shaped to the breadth of her forehead; her hair dark, wavy and fine, her skin very light." She was considered the most beautiful woman in Hawaii, and became Kamehameha's favorite wife. She would later advise him as he consolidated his rule over the Islands, and would help in reconciling jealous chiefs and holding control of the island chain for her husband's lifetime. She was later to be valued at half his kingdom.

The war in Hana continued for years. Kamehameha was there one day, in November, when runners reported breathlessly to Chief Kalani'opu'u. They told of gigantic manta rays in the night sky and great heiaus floating on the ocean. It was the tower of the great god Lono, they said. The excitement was intense, and the next morning Kalani'opu'u and Kamehameha rushed with everyone else to the shore at Wailua to stare at the strange apparitions that were indeed floating on the sea.

At the back of the crowd were several Kauai men who earlier had seen the apparitions, on their own island. They warned the people that these were not the heiaus of Lono but no one listened. Men, women, and children, commoners and chiefs, flocked unheeding to the beach. Carrying baby pigs, sugar cane, taro, breadfruit and sweet potatos, they pushed off through the surf in outriggers awash with food. Girls jumped from canoes halfway out and swam to the great hulls of the heiaus that sat still in the long ocean swells, and grasped hanging rigging to pull themselves aboard. The clamoring natives surrounded the ships in such great numbers that the strange white gods with wrinkled skin and angular heads were forced to push many back into the sea. It was impossible for all to get aboard.

Once on board, the Hawaiians stared at their visitors in astonishment. The gods wore triangular shapes on their heads, stood on narrow, covered feet, and smoke spouted from their mouths like Pele's fires. They spoke in a strange high-pitched language "like the trilling of the o-o bird," according to one memory of the time.

Kamehameha had taken the precaution of loading many canoes with black slingstones from Waianapanapa, but this proved unnecessary. When Kamehameha saw that there was no likelihood of a fight, he flattened his hair down with paste and prepared to escort Chief Kalani'opu'u to the larger of the two ships, now about three miles offshore.

The floating temples with "sails like a stingray" and caves in the side with shining holes behind, were the ships of Captain James Cook, the *Resolution* and the *Discovery*, more than two years out of England on their third Pacific voyage of exploration. Cook had dropped anchor in deep water off Maui's north shore on the calm morning of November 26, 1778. It was almost a year after Cook had briefly visited Kauai and then continued on through the Bering Strait in his unsuccessful search for a northwest passage. With the approach of winter, Captain Cook had returned to map the newly discovered islands and replenish his depleted stores. In two months he would sail into Kealakekua Bay on Hawaii Island and die at the hands of hostile natives.

When Kalani'opu'u and Kamehameha came alongside the *Discovery*, they were carefully lifted on board and escorted down a narrow gangway to Captain Cook's cabin. One of the natives in the chiefs' party caused considerable discussion among the ship's officers as he passed. At his waist were two daggers made of painted iron and shaped like skewers. The native held his two forefingers across each other in a sign of the cross and pointed to the land. The officers could not escape the impression that other white men had arrived earlier. Perhaps the Spaniards, sailing their gold-laden galleons across the trackless Pacific from Manila to Acapulco had been shipwrecked decades before on the rugged Maui shore.

Chief Kalani'opu'u presented Cook with two small hogs and his great feather cloak and after exchanging pleasantries, returned to shore, leaving Kamehameha and several retainers aboard. Kamehameha's double outrigger was secured astern.

Master William Bligh of the *Resolution* assigned men to bargain with the eager Hawaiians. Fruit and vegetables were obtained in great quantities for a few nails and simple iron tools—all that Cook's men had to trade with. The sailors refused to accept hogs of less than sixty pounds, and when the natives realized that they could not

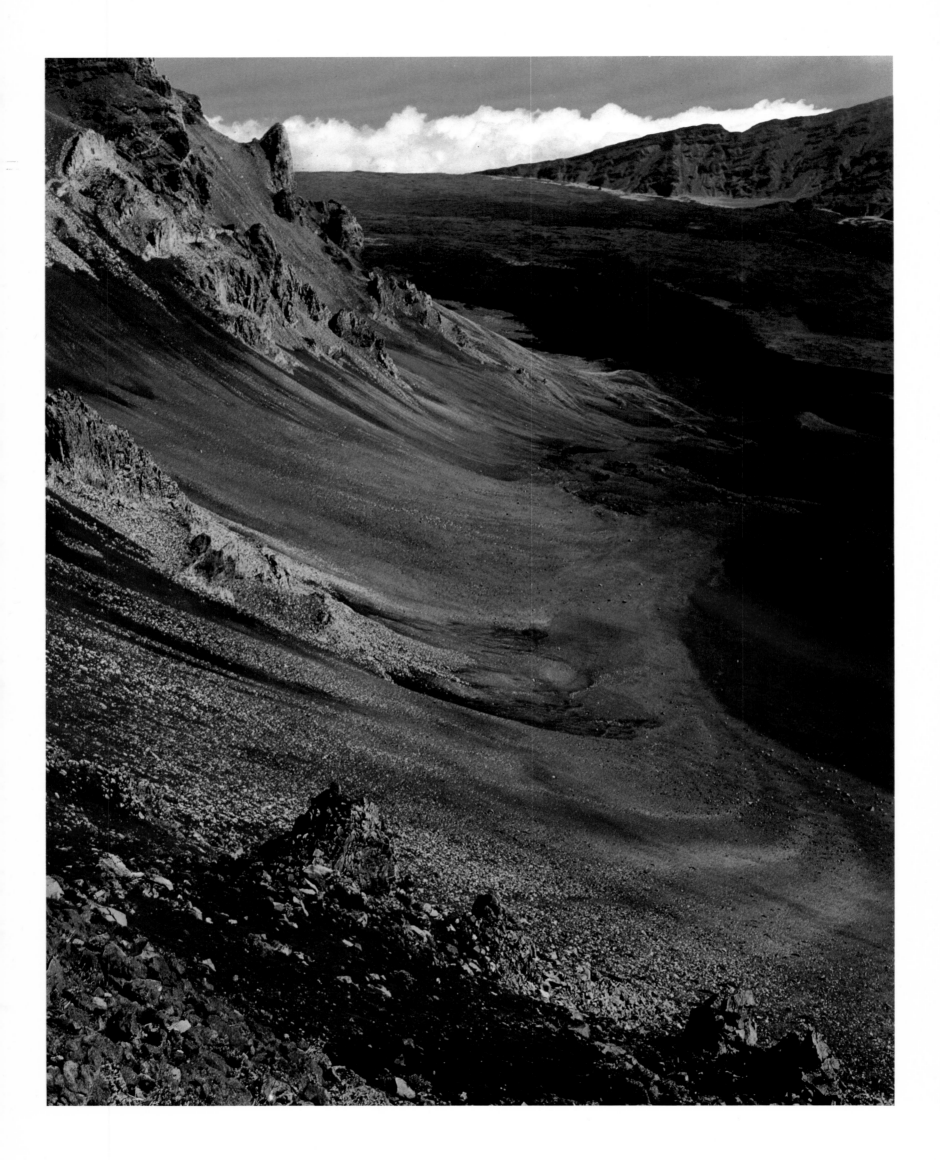

bargain for squealing piglets, they paddled back to shore and found larger animals.

In the rush to trade, some swam miles in the open ocean with breadfruit and taro in their hands and remained in the water while striking a bargain. One swimmer was trailed by a shark. Upon seeing it, the man turned around and frightened the shark away by striking it on the head with his fists. Hawaiians nearby took little notice except to glance around to assure themselves that the swimmer was safe.

It was a festive scene of noise and confusion, the laughter on ship and in the water mingled with excited. shouts in strange languages. Some Hawaiians swam the ship's length to measure it, and others stood on deck with arms stretched out in amazement. When a pet cat fell overboard from the *Discovery* it was picked up two miles astern by natives who were rewarded with an iron adz by the ship's officers, who admired their honesty.

Women were forbidden on board by Captain Cook in his effort to prevent the spread of disease, but good intentions were overwhelmed by the obvious desire of the Hawaiian girls to grant favors. They dared crew members to refuse them as they joined the Hana men dancing on deck, singing and enjoying immensely the most trivial things that presented themselves.

Cook's men soon departed the islands, but not the same set of islands they had first touched on. When the first alien seamen stepped on Hawaiian sand, a great change began. Before that event—an event that could not have seemed dark to Kamehameha or his followers, its import glimpsed, briefly, only by Cook—Hawaii had been almost a paradise. There was a brutal kapu system, but measles, flu, and syphilis were unknown. Sleeping naked on lauhala mats in the warm Hawaiian night was pleasant before mosquitoes, scorpions, disease-bearing rats, cockroaches, and centipedes were introduced by exploring white men. Most of the pests would be brought in by accident, but some of them on purpose. The larvae of mosquitoes were released deliberately in island waters when frustrated crewmen of the *Wellington*, out of San Blas, Mexico, dumped their water casks in anger because native girls were prevented from swimming out to their ship. Deliberate or not, the European touch was fatal. The dirty gray sails of European ships were harbingers of a new age, the ships vehicles for a new ecology that would make Hawaiian village life a miserable existence.

The coming of white men was to affect Kamehameha's fortunes more than those of any other Hawaiian. It was not Cook's first visit to Maui, however, or the second visit by La Pérouse, but a third visit that would help fulfill the prophecies made of Kamehameha and justify the comet that announced his birth.

The arrival of Jean François de Galaup de la Pérouse, the first explorer to set foot on Maui, was of small moment. La Pérouse anchored his ships, *Boussole* and *Astrolabe*, off East Maui and stepped ashore at the bay named in his honor. He had sailed by Kipahulu the day before, hoping for a landing, as his water ration was reduced to a single bottle a day. He wrote in his journal that he and his men "beheld water falling in cascades from the mountains, and running in streams to the sea after having watered the habitations of the natives, which are so numerous that a space of three or four leagues may be taken for a single village. The trees which crowned the mountains and the verdure of the banana plants that surrounded the habitations produced inexpressible charms to our senses, but the sea beat upon the coast with the utmost violence and kept us in the situation of Tantalus, desiring and devouring with our eyes what was impossible for us to attain."

La Pérouse sailed away and it was not until 1790 that another ship visited Maui, the *Eleanora*, commanded by Captain Simon Metcalfe, an American fur trader. In the course of the *Eleanora*'s visit, some Hawaiians stole a longboat from her, killing the sailor who guarded it and breaking up the boat for its iron. In retaliation, Metcalfe killed with grapeshot more than one hundred Hawaiians who sat in canoes about his ship.

News of the incident spread rapidly. Natives across the channel on Hawaii Island soon learned of it, and led by a Hawaii chief whom Metcalfe had flogged earlier, they determined to take revenge. Within days, they spotted the innocent sloop *Fair American*, captained by Metcalfe's son, close inshore at north Kona. Assaulting the small vessel from outrigger canoes, they killed all but one of the five-man crew, drowned young Metcalfe, and enthusiastically looted below decks. The wounded survivor, Isaac Davis, swam ashore through the pounding surf of north Kona. He would later become an *aikane*, or companion-servant, of Kamehameha.

Unaware of the *Fair American*'s capture, Captain Metcalfe's *Eleanora* put in at Hawaii for fresh food and water. A lone seaman went ashore for a day of liberty, and learned of the smaller ship's fate. Kamehameha refused him permission to return to his ship for fear that he would tell Metcalfe. Kamehameha did not want on Hawaii Island a repetition of the Maui massacre. The seaman, John Young,

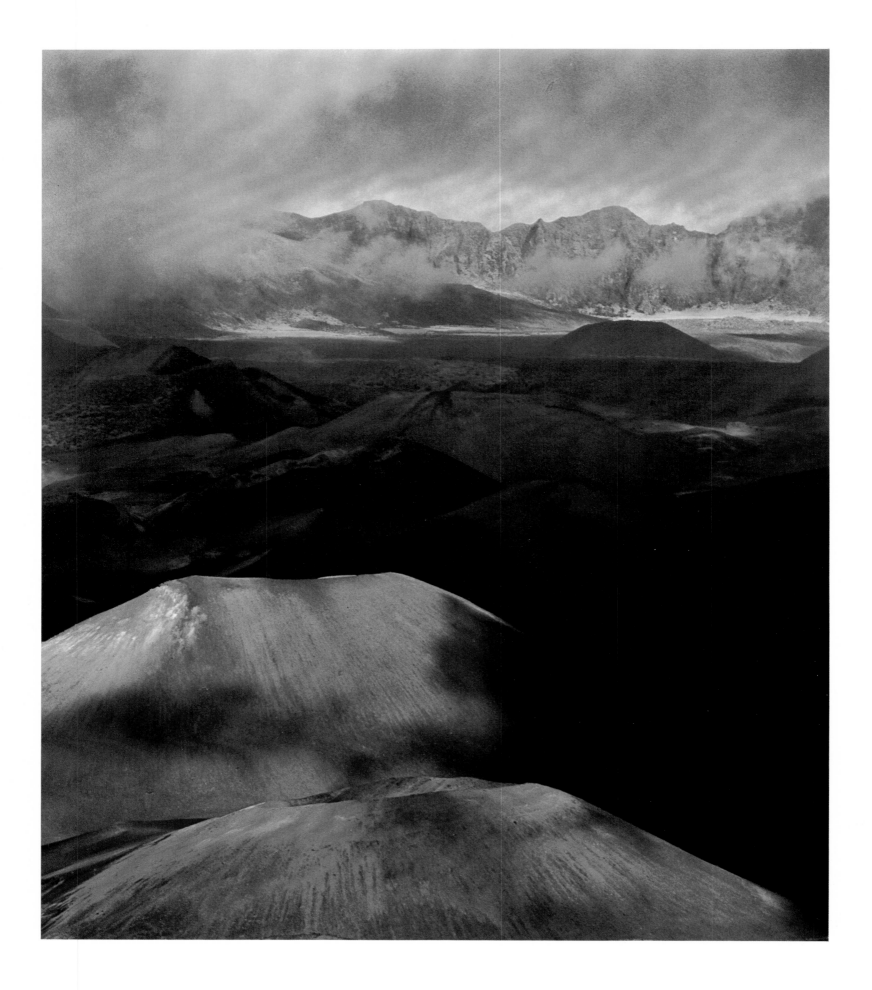

was asked as Isaac Davis had been to become Kamehameha's *aikane*. The *Eleanora*, after tacking back and forth waiting the seaman's return, sailed away in the gathering darkness, noting a deserter in her log.

Kamehameha's acquisition of the sloop *Fair American* was important to his conquest of the Islands. With the sloop came muskets, knives, powder, cannon, and most providentially, the men to use them in battle. Watching Young and Davis shoot at some distance a pig and wild cock, Kamehameha was delighted, realizing that he now controlled the weapons necessary for subjugation of the other islands. He sent messengers to the ruling chiefs of his own island, demanding canoes and men to mount an expedition against the ruling chief of Maui.

The invasion that followed came before Kamehameha had secured complete loyalty on his own island, but was the first step in his conquest. He sailed for Maui fully prepared to set up court with his counselors, chiefs, the younger relatives and sons of lesser chiefs, and a loyal army of warriors eager to fight for the great Kamehameha. His great fleet of canoes landed on every stone beach along the Hana coast, and the battle called *Kawa'anui*, the many canoes, began. The defending forces were vanquished in the first skirmish, and Kamehameha stepped ashore in the early evening, declaring himself ruler of Maui, and built shelters on the spot. His red feather war god, Kuka'ilimoku, was displayed prominently on a stone altar.

The next day Kamehameha pursued the fleeing enemy along the Kiha-a-Piilani Highway and put them to death when they became exhausted on the steep ascents. He marched on swiftly to Wailuku, where the forces of the Maui chiefs resisted for two days, fighting resolutely until Young and Davis brought up their cannon and slaughtered the defenders at the narrow entrance to Iao Valley. The frightened survivors scrambled up the cliffs to escape, but the cannon were hauled closer and the fleeing men shot off the high palis. The battle went down in Hawaiian history as *Kapaniwai*, "the damming of the waters," for so many were killed that their bodies choked Iao stream.

With his wife Ka-ahumanu and his entourage of chiefs, Kamehameha moved on to Molokai, landing without resistance, but learning there that his home districts of Kohala and Waipio had been ravaged in his absence. "While I have been seeking new children," Kamehameha said, "my first-born have been abandoned." He returned to Hawaii Island to put down the rebellious chiefs before resuming his conquest of all the islands, the conquest that established the Hawaiian Kingdom.

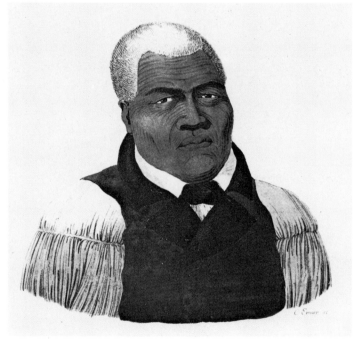

Kamehameha

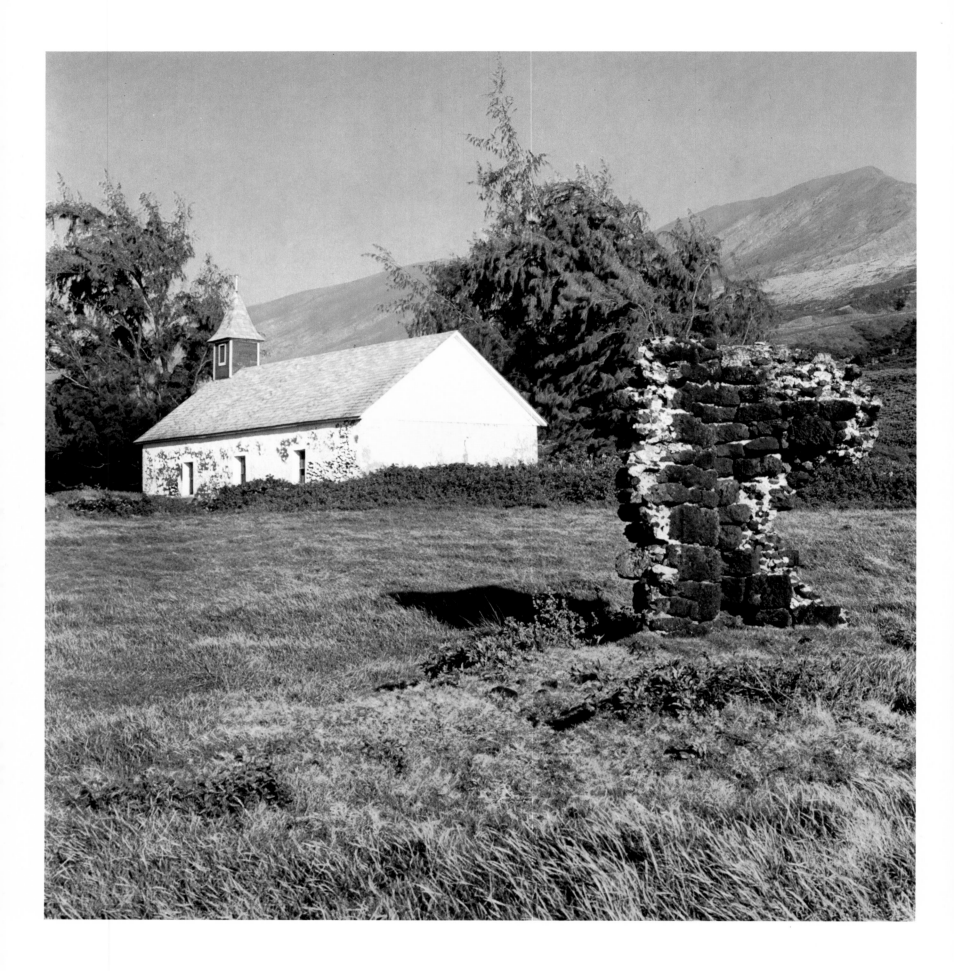

4. Missionaries

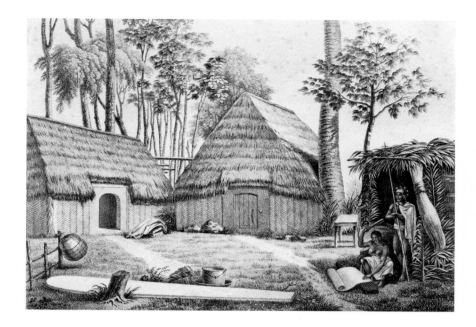

THE FIRST American missionary company, dedicated to the abolishment of heathen rites in Hawaii, was several weeks out of Boston in the tiny brig *Thaddeus* when King Liholiho announced the abandonment of the Hawaiian kapu system. Kamehameha's favorite wife, Ka-ahumanu, who had become a huge woman—and Prime Minister of the Hawaiian Kingdom—after her husband's death, had encouraged his successor Liholiho in his efforts to end the archaic prohibitions. She publicly ate with the new king, and in other ways demonstrated the emancipation of Hawaiian women.

When the Congregational missionaries arrived in 1820, the idols were already burned and the heathen priests repudiated by their own chiefs. It was not difficult for the missionaries to fill the void in a society temporarily without moral law and order, and Christianity was proclaimed the new religion without major opposition.

The Reverend Hiram Bingham, lately of Boston, saw little in the Islands to commend, however. The pili-thatched huts, perched on smooth stone platforms and ideally suited to the warm Hawaiian weather, did not please the Reverend. They could not be "washed, scoured, polished, or painted to good purpose or made suitable for good furniture." He reviled the old Hawaiian culture for its "abominable priests," and the populace for the "appearance of destitution, degradation and barbarism, among the chattering, and almost naked savages, whose heads and feet and much of their sunburnt swarthy skins were bare." He found little to compare favorably with New England and considered the whole scene "appalling," though by almost every measure the Hawaiian commoner enjoyed a life considerably richer than the European peasant or pieceworker in the contemporary industrial ghetto of New England.

Long after most of the other islands had abandoned the ancient kapus, the people of Hana in their isolation still spoke cautiously of the *kahunas*, the priests who whispered in the night, planning vengeance on kapu violators. It was eight years before the first group of missionaries visited East Maui, and when the resident missionary and his family arrived in 1837, the natives looked with interest at the first white woman and baby seen in Hana.

The Reverend and Mrs. Daniel Toll Conde had spent several months in Lahaina studying the Hawaiian language before embarking on the small native coastal schooner *Hooikaika*. In the crowd of naked passengers who slept and ate on deck, Mrs. Conde huddled with her three-month-old baby, on a large straw-filled mattress, afraid to let the infant be touched by the "filthy" Hawaiians and unable to eat during the night and two days of the voyage. She stepped ashore at Hana weak and fearful, walking shakily with her husband to her new home, a primitive grass hut that topped a slight rise above Hana Bay. The Conde's Hawaiian home was like all the other village huts, with a single, low entrance and floor of black beach pebbles covered with several layers of woven lauhala mats, soft and springy underfoot. It had been built by the Hana people for the new priest of their new religion. The Condes couldn't wait to leave it for something stuffier.

The native women were fascinated by the white baby, but Mrs. Conde repulsed all attempts by the heathen to take the baby in their arms. The heathen, nevertheless, brought food of all kinds to the famished newcomers, and soon the empty hut was filled with smells of taro, bananas, sweet potatoes, breadfruit, and poi.

On Sunday, a large shelter of lauhala thatch became the Hana church, and an eager congregation of noisy Hawaiians, covered scantily in tapa, squatted with upturned faces and waited for the service to begin. Conde stood between two groups of Hawaiians, separated by sexes, and haltingly read his first sermon in Hawaiian.

Hui O Aloha Church, Kaupo

During the following week, Conde proceeded to make his grass shack livable, cutting high doors and windows and dividing with a mat partition the single room into living and sleeping areas. He found some rough boards to floor the living room and carpeted them with lauhala mats while curious natives crowded around to watch. They helped unpack the odd articles that Conde had brought all the way from Boston—a rocking chair, bedstead, table, and bureau. After arranging the furniture suitably, the Condes invited the natives in for a visit, eight or ten at a time, not forgetting to detain them with a few words about The Saviour before letting in the next group.

Hawaiians came from as far as Kipahulu and Ko'olau to marvel at the furniture and the strangers who sat in chairs. They came from Hamoa in droves and crowded into the tiny hut. The windows, cut so carefully by Reverend Conde to allow light and air to enter, were obstructed from dawn to dusk by dark faces peering in for a glimpse of the white mother and child.

As time passed and Sunday congregations grew larger, Conde began to feel that he was succeeding. He was teaching the basic principles of Christianity and Western Civilization with earnestness and perseverance, completely isolated from the companionship of fellow missionaries. Reverend Conde and his wife labored together teaching school, visiting the sick, vaccinating against smallpox, and attempting to heal with limited knowledge and medicine. They helped natives register their house sites and taro patches by filling out required forms and corresponding with government authorities in Honolulu. The Hawaiians responded with loyalty and devotion to the Christian ministry. When Reverend Conde's grass hut burned to the ground, a new convert, the owner of a nearby house that recently had been completed, immediately offered it to the destitute missionary family.

Conde found the Hawaiians "profoundly ignorant; their intellects exceedingly obtuse, and as to moral sense they seemed quite destitute of it. Their homes too were mere hovels thatched with grass, low, contracted and filthy. They lived mostly in a nude state. Not a garment of foreign manufacture was worn by male or female. But they were very approachable, kind and tractable."

These kind and tractable people danced and played too much. Conde and the other pastors from New England considered the hula disgusting and a moral menace that should be vigorously condemned. Hawaiians were reminded every Sunday that the hula and other of the last vestiges of pagan ceremonies must be abolished. The missionaries stopped ti-leaf sliding and surfing at Keanini, objecting to the impropriety of "men and women surfing together in scanty costumes," and to the betting that took place on long rides. Sports wasted time that could be better spent in productive labor and learning the Saviour's word. The missionaries introduced a new kapu system, prohibiting in the name of God all dancing, feasting, music, nakedness, gambling, drinking, games, and adultery.

Except for chiefs of high rank there had been little more to a marriage ceremony than exchanges of mutual devotion. Either party could end the arrangement by simply going off to another house, and was restrained from doing so only by a general sentiment against changing mates too frequently. A man was free to have two or more wives, and a wife two or more husbands. Governor Hoapili of Maui set an example for change in 1823 when he married chiefess Kalekua in a Christian ceremony. Six years later, on the urging of the American Mission Board, King Kamehameha III decreed that "it is not proper that one man have two wives." Afterward Hoapili forbade men and women to live together without benefit of Christian ceremony. Offenders were punished by being made to work on a public road.

The new law required each man with more than one wife to keep his favorite and discard the rest. This was a hardship on the discarded women, who found it difficult to find shelter and food, but there were punishments for those who failed to comply. A man caught for the second time in adultery, for example, was required to "pay three hogs to the husband of his paramour, and three to the governor, who shall set apart a portion for the King, if not hogs then something else of equal value."

The old heiau at the foot of Ka'uiki Head, first constructed by Umi-a-Liloa's warriors, was dismantled on Conde's orders and the once-sacred stones carried by Christian converts to the site of a new temple of worship. The best divers collected coral for lime from the depths of Hana Bay, and a dozen of the most skillful church members began to lay the foundation for a permanent church. Natives dragged ohia timbers from the wet mountains above Hana for rafters and beams, and supervised by Conde cut roof plates to the proper size.

A discharged sailor, skilled in carpentry, wandered into Hana. Reverend Conde thanked God, and immediately hired the man to frame the high-pitched roof. While the sailor worked, Hana's weighty women, now completely covered in colorful muumuus from head to foot, prepared great lauhala mats to cover the cold mortar floor. Conde himself built the pulpit of Hawaiian hardwood. A heavy bronze bell was mounted in a small belfry.

Reverend Conde, who had preached his first service to fourteen curious neophytes, was by 1841 sometimes offering his sermon to three thousand people. The great native congregation, without musical instruments or hymnals, sprang to their feet when the preacher called out "Nu Oli," and they responded like a great organ in Hawaiian, "Good news, good news, a wonderful message. The news of salvation, come from heaven." It must have been gratifying to Reverend Conde, and when he left Hana after eleven years there he must have felt that he had succeeded.

The discovery of gold in California the year after Conde left gave the missionaries their first great problem. Sutter's find immediately made the Hawaiian Islands important economically. Ships from San Francisco docked in increasing numbers at Kahului on Maui for cargoes of vegetables and fresh produce to supply the hordes of miners that were sweeping into the Sierra Nevada foothills. Coastal steamers calling at Hana did a thriving trade for yams, arrowroot, and bananas. Hana's wild sugar cane found a ready market in the Chinese laborers working California mines, and Hawaiian families were soon neglecting not only their taro patches, but also the Christian family life so carefully organized by the Hana church. The natives purchased what they wanted and neglected to pray. Regular church members began to absent themselves from meetings, and began to commit what the missionaries regarded as "overt acts of sin and iniquity" with their new wealth.

The desire for manufactured products that had been encouraged by the missionaries was now working against them. Money was spent frivolously, with little regard for consequences. Gambling flourished. Civilization had suddenly come full turn for the men of God, and the decline of religious interest became their great concern.

Another blow to the Protestant missionaries was the arrival of French Catholics. The Catholics were protected in their work by Oahu's Governor Boki, who thus became a rival of Ka-ahumanu, the champion of Protestants. Chiefs loyal to Ka-ahumanu considered Protestantism the state religion, and made several attempts to banish priests and punish the growing number of Catholic converts for idolatry.

Hana's small Protestant group at first ignored the religious interlopers, fully expecting the Hawaiians to reject the "false" doctrine. But Helio Koaeloa, a Catholic layman born in Wailua village, became particularly bothersome and converted hundreds of natives in the rugged Kipahulu area. After his own acceptance of the catechism, Helio traveled to all sections of Maui, zealously spreading the faith. Reverend Conde's mission was alarmed, and forbade natives to attend Catholic services.

When the Hana mission learned that several women converted by Helio were holding private Catholic prayer meetings in a small hut near Kaupo's Protestant church, the mission informed the Wailuku judge, who immediately sent police to arrest the culprits. The native police dragged the Catholic converts from their homes, assembled the small group, tied them together with sennit, and started them on the ninety-mile return trip to Wailuku in central Maui.

As the forced march began, word quickly traveled ahead along the Kiha-a-Piilani Highway. Soon at every turn small groups of Catholics were gathering to profess their faith and be tied with the Kaupo converts. As the proud procession passed through Kipahulu, Wailua, Pu'uiki and Hamoa, it grew steadily in size. The new Catholics, dressed in their best, draped leis upon the prisoners, and fell in step. The procession continued on, enjoying the bountiful hospitality of communities along the trail, sometimes remaining two or three days in the same village, holding prayer meetings at every opportunity and bringing in new members at Wailua, Keanae, and Heleo. The procession was in a carnival mood when it finally neared Wailuku. It had been more than a month on the trail and had grown a hundredfold.

When the Catholic neophytes, still tied together, crowded noisily into the tiny Wailuku courthouse, the judge took one look at the crowd of demonstrators, thought of the consequences of prosecuting them, and promptly dismissed the case.

Helio and his brother Petero decided to return along the route of the march to encourage their new converts and enroll still more. There was now widespread native support for the Catholic faith, and soon there were many plans for Catholic chapels along the Kiha-a-Piilani Highway. With an old heiau for foundation, the first small Catholic church was built at the entrance to Kipahulu Valley.

5. Sugar

IN 1849, Hana's first sugar works was erected a short distance from Ka'uiki Head. It was a modest beginning—several grass shacks sheltering four large cast-iron try pots purchased from a whaleship and set high enough on a foundation of lava rocks to permit building a wood fire beneath. Hana's first plantation, sixty acres of cane, was planted nearby, and the cane was harvested, stripped of leaves, and fed by hand into a wooden mill worked by four yoke of cattle.

The plantation manager was a seaman named George Wilfong, the second officer of a whaler out of New England. Wilfong arrived in Lahaina the year the plantation began operating. There, on learning of the discovery of gold in California, he had purchased his discharge to try his luck in the Sierra gold fields. While waiting for passage, Wilfong roomed with the Lahaina Police Magistrate, who milled cane and sold sugar on the side. By the time his ship arrived, Wilfong had become more infatuated with dreams of sugar than dreams of gold, and sailed to Hana to manage the new plantation. He took over the primitive mills, stock, and caneland, and began to learn the sugar business.

Of his arrival Wilfong later said, "I was much pleased with the place, the plant cane was very promising and wild cane everywhere." The wild juices were easily converted into sugar, and without prior knowledge of testing procedures, Wilfong judged the strength of the juice by taste and appearance. When the syrup looked good to him, he shipped the product to Lahaina where it always sold for a good price. Hana seemed to be a natural place for sugar to grow.

Learning the business by himself, Wilfong saved the usual $300 fee for lessons in sugar boiling. When his hired sugar boiler died, Wilfong took on the job and, following the procedures he had watched so carefully, made his own "strike." In 1852 he purchased an iron grinding mill, but became so exasperated with the man sent out from Honolulu to assemble it that he fired him, and with the help of a Hawaiian blacksmith, completed construction himself. He imported a mason to put up the chimney and together they set up a chain of five boiling kettles.

A primitive centrifuge was installed to separate the molasses from the raw sugar. Powered by four men through wheel and belt, the rapidly whirling machine was a great curiosity to the Hawaiians. Wilfong wrote that "sometimes a hundred or more natives came to see it run, the school boys would come every afternoon and run the machine until night without pay, and would dispute their turn to run it, they would make it hum."

Relying on his experience as a whaleship officer, Wilfong hired local natives as "shipped" labor. He signed them up to work his plantation as he would have signed sailors, requiring the Hawaiians to enter into a formal contract for as long as ten years, and to do a certain kind of plantation work for so many hours a day. To attract Hawaiians away from their village life he often would pay a considerable portion of their salaries in advance, sometimes as much as $150. The Hawaiian often drew all the advance he could get and promptly squandered it at Wilfong's general store in Hana. Unable to receive more pay, the Hawaiian asked for credit, and soon was working out endless days that neither paid anything nor reduced his years of indenture. Baffled by the system, many fled to plantations in central Maui where they might "ship on" again and receive another advance. And there was another alternative for the Hawaiian worker. "When his needs became very pressing," an early plantation report states, "he would endeavor to secure a fresh advance by shipping over again where he was, for a new term on top of the balance of the old; and he would do this with the utmost equanimity, as often the master would consent, until he became so hopelessly involved that nothing but death could be expected to set him free."

Under this system the indentured Hawaiian was quite reluctant to work, and took advantage of every possible excuse. He was always ready to plead illness, and the death of even the most distant relative required his immediate attendance. Wilfong arrested many workers who habitually failed to appear at the sugar house, charging them with *haalele hana*—quitting work. They were duly convicted, fined and ordered to return to the mill. They could not pay the fine, of course, so Wilfong paid it for them and charged it to their account, to be worked out along with everything else.

A law was passed requiring the indentured plantation laborer to put in two days time for every day he lost in jail for haalele hana. This was added to the end of his contract and worsened the relationship between the

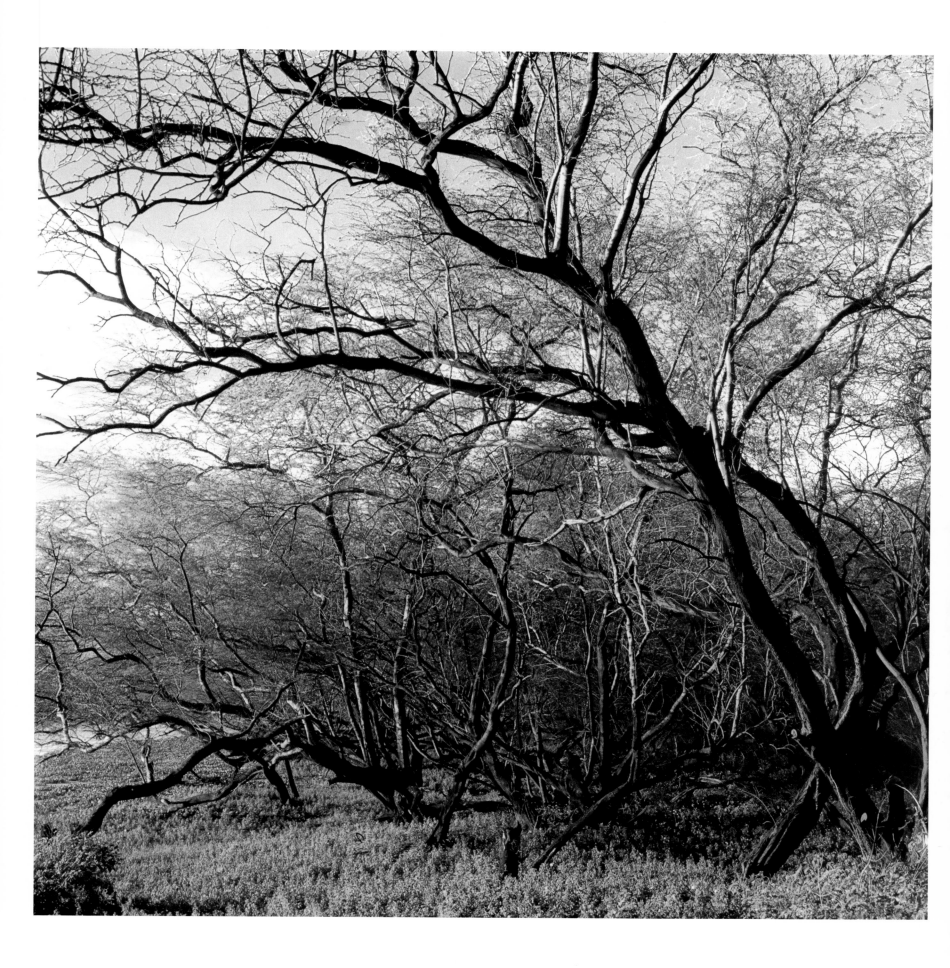

Hawaiians and their employers. The natives became discouraged and abandoned their jobs in large numbers. They saw little advantage in working from dawn to dusk under a system that defied understanding. Many Hawaiians shipped out for the gold fields—so many that laws were passed forbidding natives from emigrating to California without permission from the King.

The planters' labor problems in Hana, and elsewhere in Hawaii, quickly became so serious that contract labor laws were passed. In 1852 the first Chinese laborers began arriving in Hana, but they proved unreliable as field hands and many left the plantation to become merchants and artisans on their own. Wages of three dollars a month were little incentive to stay.

The Hawaiians of Hana, now forced by threats and jailing to work in the sugar fields, or enticed into working long hours for the manufactured articles displayed in Wilfong's general store, often fled to remote villages, but new recruits continued to arrive from Hamoa and beyond to build their bamboo homes near the mill. Neither the recruited Hawaiians nor the original residents who stayed were able to grow their own taro, and they became further dependent upon Wilfong when he began to sell cheap pounded poi at his store. The poi, and the salt salmon that was occasionally distributed with it, all wrapped in ti leaves, was to ensure a good turnout for work. Hardtack biscuits soon were added, then dried beef, and the Hawaiians had acquired a new diet.

The caneworker's job was arduous and monotonous. He toiled from dawn to darkness, and only heavy rain and Sunday church services offered relief. There was little leisure time, even for family life. The harvested cane, stripped of leaves, had to be hauled in from the fields on muleback and piled in the mill yard. The iron crusher, driven by cattle yoked into teams and plodding a tight circle, received the long stalks of cane, pulled from a pile in the yard and carefully fed between the rollers by hand. From the mill, a thin stream of foaming juice ran in an open trough to the boiling house a short distance away.

In the dim interior of the boiling house, a native kept the pots boiling continuously over roaring wood fires while his sweating partner swept scum off the bubbling juice with a long wooden paddle. Clouds of smoke and steam rose to the open ceiling, and the steam condensed on the tin roof, falling back as large drops of sugar-sweetened rain.

As the boiling juice slowly became thicker, it was bailed over from one pot to the next until finally, in the last pot, it was tested. A native dipped a long thin *hau* stick into the pot, raised it, and let the stick drip into a large opihi shell full of water. He rubbed the sample between his fingers and held it up to the light to judge whether the juice had cooked sufficiently to "strike." When he was satisfied, the last pot was promptly emptied into cooling barrels and allowed to remain, sometimes for weeks, until the sugar had grained up from the bottom. The dark brown syrup was then poured into tubs and carried to the centrifuge for separation, and the dry, raw sugar packed into small wooden kegs with a heavy wooden pounder, and stored until sufficient quantities were available for profitable shipment. The remaining molasses was poured into a large wood tank outside the boiling house.

Before the plantation life had become the traditional life for the Hawaiians of Hana, Wilfong's mill burned to the ground. The fire destroyed more than fifty tons of sugar and burst the molasses tank, almost drowning several workers who were attempting to move it away from the burning buildings. Wilfong attempted to rebuild, for there was still a fine crop growing in the fields, but he was rebuffed by the merchants in Honolulu, who then considered sugar a poor business risk. They refused him credit, and persuaded him to give up the idea, reminding him that the sugar plantation at Haiku had already failed and been abandoned. Wilfong took his stock of goods and opened up a general store across Alenuihaha Channel. When that too failed, he returned to the sea.

The carefully planted cane fields of Hana grew wild again, and weeds soon covered the mill. Many natives, released by default from years of indentured labor, returned to village life and grew taro again as their forefathers had. Some used their new agricultural knowledge to raise truck crops to sell in Kahului. Many returned to the church. For almost ten years the abandoned Hana cane bent untouched to the harsh channel winds. It was not until 1864 and the arrival of two Danish brothers, August and Oscar Unna, that the sugar business returned to Hana.

August Unna had fought as an artillery lieutenant in the Danish army during the Schleswig-Holstein war, and had worked as a butcher in Lahaina for several years before moving to Hana. Like so many others before him, he began sugar planting without experience. Seeing the possibility of great wealth in sugar, he enlisted the aid of his brother, and together they were able to raise $47,000 to establish a new Hana plantation. Their enterprise was successful and the brothers acquired an island-wide reputation in the industry, for many of the innovations in early sugar technology originated in Hana. August Unna was active in the newly established Royal Hawaiian Agricultural Society, and experimented with some of the first imported labor on his Hana plantation. He became a

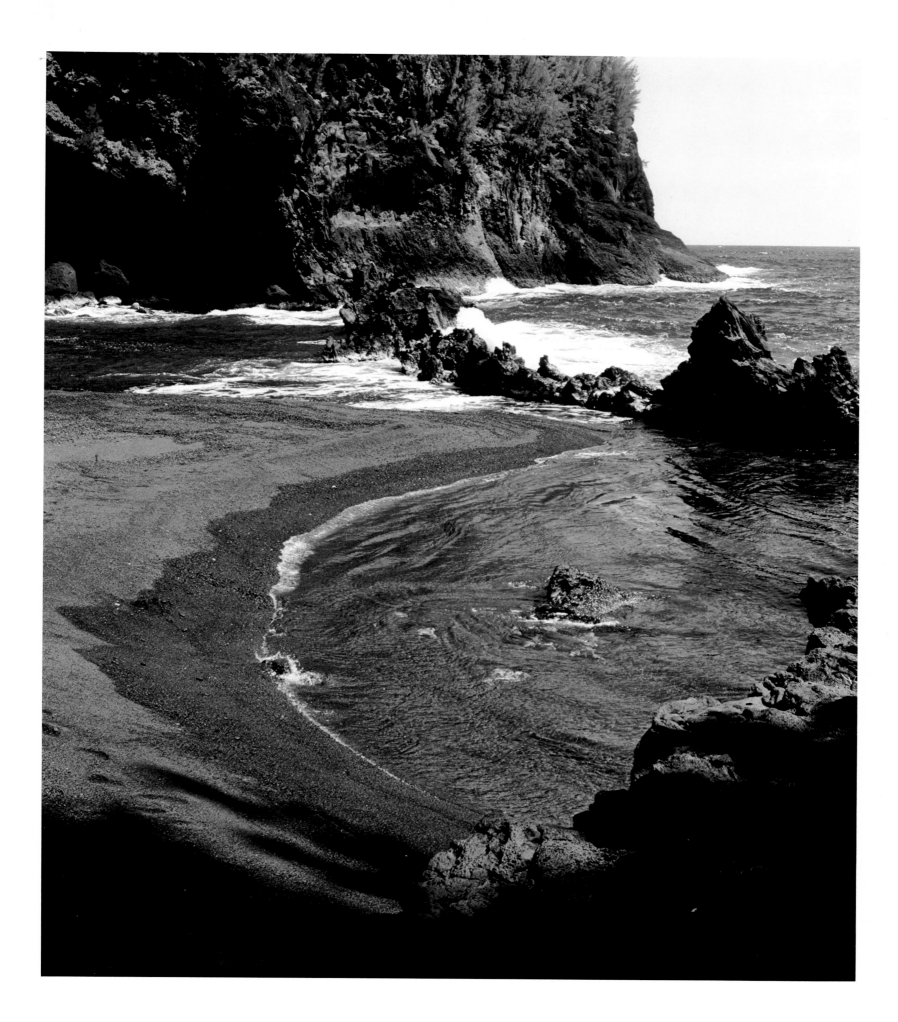

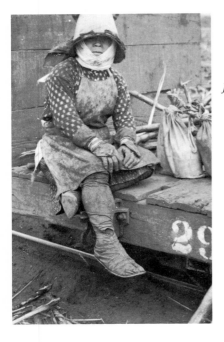

Japanese Sugar Worker

member of the planters' committee that drafted alien-labor contracts.

Labor was still a serious problem in Hana. Few Hawaiians returned to work in the mill, preferring to fish and till their own land. Occasionally they would help out during peak harvesting months to earn a few dollars, but nothing could get them back in the fields or the mill for more than a few weeks' time. The attempt to import Chinese field hands had failed, so the planters turned to Japan. In 1868 the first Japanese laborers, both men and women, arrived in Hana with three-year contracts and the desire to return rich and successful to their homeland. They were for the most part agricultural workers from southern Japan, an adventurous group anxious to improve their lot. Plantation life was a rude shock.

Posted proclamations reminded the new laborers that the plantation was run like a ship, with the manager's authority absolute. Their new homes were crude dormitory shacks, many of them constructed by local natives who refused to work in the sugar fields themselves. There were rules for everything, for the work day as well as for worship and sleep:

"Laborers are expected to be industrious and docile and obedient to their overseers. Laborers are expected to be regular and cleanly in their personal habits, to retire to rest and rise at the appointed hours. No fires will be allowed after 6:30 P.M. and no lights after 8:30 P.M. Every laborer is required to be in bed at 8:30 P.M. and to rise at 5:00 A.M. During the hours appointed for rest, no talking is permitted or any noise calculated to disturb those wishing to rest. Gambling, fast riding, and leaving the plantation without permission are strictly forbidden."

Workers were fined one quarter of their wages if late for work and were expected on the job before daylight to work a ten-hour day. There was a twenty-five cent fine for smoking on the job or stealing a stalk of sugar cane, and the value of any missing or broken tools was taken out of the eighteen to twenty dollars a month the laborer received as wages. Management provided free housing, medical care, and the Hana general store, where much of the money paid out by the plantation found its way back in the inflated prices received for manufactured goods. But half of the Japanese worker's wages, a princely sum by Japanese standards, was deposited in Honolulu banks and awaited his triumphant return to Japan.

In the early morning hours, men and women were herded into the mill yard by white field *lunas* who, according to one frightened immigrant writing home, "looked like demons or terrible gods as they rode by on horseback with their long snakelike leather whips." The laborers were marched to the fields, where they worked steadily, stopping only at midday to eat their daily fare of rice, boiled turnips, and meat. After each day's work they returned to poorly ventilated rooms and wood plank beds with straw mats, where as many as half a dozen men and women slept together.

As a result of numerous complaints, the Japanese government dispatched a special envoy to Hawaii for an investigation of working conditions, and an amicable settlement was reached with the Hawaiian government in Honolulu. Rule changes provided that everyone would be paid for holidays and rainy weather. Strict house rules were relaxed and there was to be no more whipping of workers in the fields.

August Unna continued to clear land for new cane. The lauhala, *ama'u* ferns, and *ha'u* thickets were burned off, twisted root systems were hacked out by hand and the soil plowed by bullocks. A new mill was steadily expanded with modern machinery designed in Honolulu, and each year the mill became larger and more efficient. By 1894, Hana produced 2700 tons of sugar a year.

Hana soon gained a reputation as a delightful place to visit, and Unna's new home, built in traditional New England style, became a mecca for visitors to East Maui. King Kalakaua stayed often, and shortly began constructing his own small cottage along the shore at Koali. He often stayed overnight at Unna's plantation house, bringing an army of retainers and his own chef, who took over the kitchen and prepared the elaborate continental meals enjoyed by the King. A long table was set in the dining room for almost two dozen people, and the King assumed the seat of honor, flanked on both sides of the table by

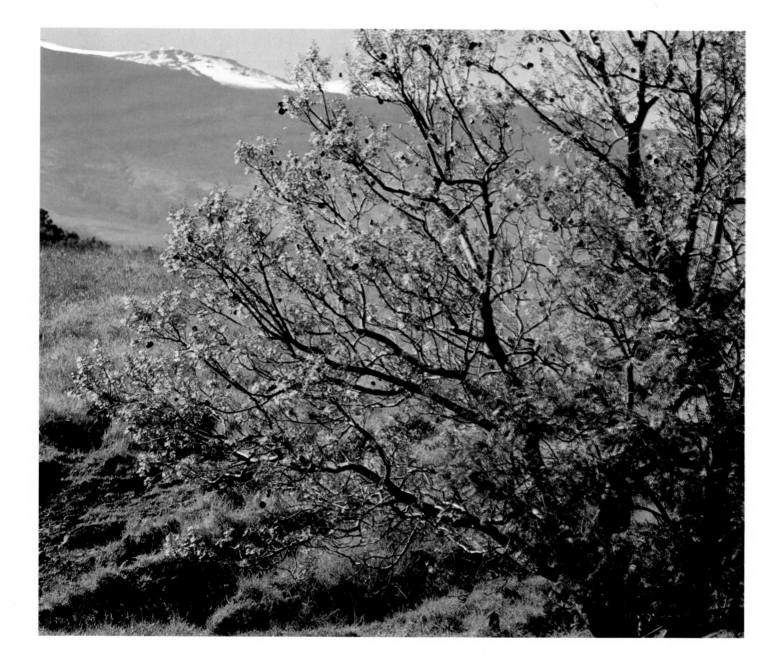

chamberlains and ministers with their Hawaiian wives. He reserved the seat at his right for the only white woman then resident in Hana, Mrs. Meta Hedemann, wife of the Danish plantation engineer. Kalakaua carved expertly, always offering the first portion to Mrs. Hedemann, then passing the platter on around the table.

The King spoke excellent English, and after dinner retired to the sitting room with Mrs. Hedemann on his arm. On his first visit he asked Mrs. Hedemann about Denmark and seemed much interested in a large photograph album of Danish sculpture. Mrs. Hedemann wrote later that she was "greatly surprised to hear him talk about some of the works, and how well he was posted on the old northern mythology."

Late in the evening of one visit, Kalakaua took Mr. Hedemann aside and said, "Now my people, the kanakas, their women, and all the hula girls will come in here, and there will be hula dancing, singing, and a generally lively and gay time. When my people get started, they sometimes get a little too lively. Of course, they do it to entertain me and my household, and it is perfectly harmless, but not exactly anything for your young wife to be at." Mr. Hedemann escorted his wife home, and Kalakaua took over Unna's vast house to play again the old games frowned upon by the Hana missionaries. For a night, Hana returned to its pagan days, the girls wildly dancing the hula, clad only in waist-high pa'us, the men drinking quantities of *okolehao*, brewed from the roasted root of the ti plant.

Princess Ruth Keelikolani was another royal visitor who came to Hana often. She was the half sister of two Kamehamehas and was once considered a possible heir to the throne. A proud woman, she had great feeling for Hawaiian tradition, avoided foreign habits, and spoke little English. She weighed more than 300 pounds, and on visits to Hana was hoisted by block and tackle directly ashore from the coastal schooner that brought her. Too heavy for a horse, she rode reclining on a mattress in a cart drawn by four plantation bullocks. Her slow progress along the Hana road was accompanied by the yelling of drivers and the cracking of long whips, and was followed by great crowds of shouting, naked children who skipped and ran alongside. Workers in the field stopped to watch the procession and native men and women on horseback cheered on the Princess, who was too large to sit up and respond. That was Princess Ruth.

As sugar changed Maui's culture, so it changed the look of the Maui landscape. The color, smell, shape, and texture of the land was altered as plantations spread. The plains between East and West Maui, once desert that grew scarcely a blade of grass, became, with irrigation, a green land.

The very sounds of the land changed. Native lowland birds were replaced by exotics brought in by the new immigrants from China and Japan. The Chinese thrush was introduced in the early 1900's, and later the Japanese bush warbler. The tiny ricebird soon was there, its plaintive monotone call sounding across unfamiliar fields. A few native birds survived in isolated valleys and high swamps, safe from the mongooses that sugar planters had imported to rid their fields of rats, only to discover that rats foraged by night while the mongooses ate by day.

Helpful homeland friends of Japanese immigrants sent small boxes of an old Japanese delicacy, the giant African snail, and it too spread through the island, like a slow and wingless, but ravaging locust that consumed native and exotic plants with impartiality.

The look of the people changed. The Hawaiian population continued to decline, while the Oriental and European populations continued to grow. The native culture and language fell with the native trees and plants cleared for cane. As swiftly as Chinese stores appeared along the Kiha-a-Piilani Highway, Japanese shops followed, selling goods imported from the homeland and distributing publications printed in the strange calligraphy of the Orient. Portuguese followed the Japanese and invented the ukulele for the Hawaiians.

The Japanese continued to arrived in shiploads. The sugar planters who brought them profited from the cheap labor, but were criticized by the many haole residents who feared the "yellow invasion." During King Kalakaua's regime, Japanese and Chinese were prohibited as "Asiatics" from voting. The Japanese responded by establishing their own language schools and publishing the first Japanese newspaper in 1892.

One of the new Hawaiians was a young man named Nick Soon. Nick Soon's father, who in his youth had been a companion of Chinese patriot Sun Yat Sen, had moved to Hawaii and become manager of a chain of Chinese stores that stretched from Kaupo to Keanae. In some communities the Soon stores were the only shops available to the native population, and offered the only overnight rooms for travelers on the Kiha-a-Piilani Highway.

The Soon family had arrived in Hawaii with the first Chinese contract workers, and like most Chinese found little to be gained by staying on the plantation. The Chinese all left as quickly as possible. They either established small trading stores, as the Soons did, or planted rice, or

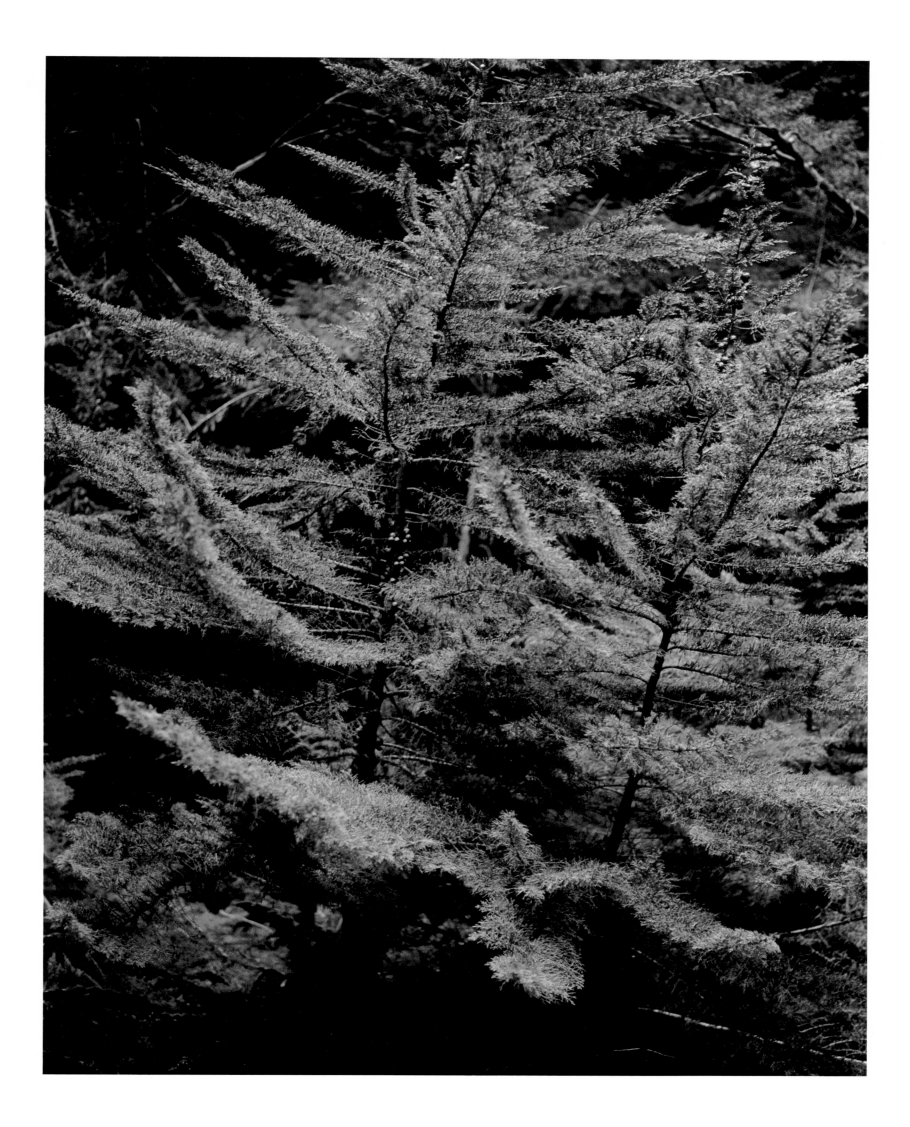

married native girls and settled down to grow taro. Chinese traditionally held ownership of land to be important, and royal land grants held by Hawaiian women married to Chinese men were seldom split up by the sugar industry's land agents. The Soons were among those who acquired property, and they prospered.

One of Nick Soon's early tasks was to meet the boats that brought stock to the Look Kee store at Kaupo, the

strated a model airplane that flew almost the length of the Kipahulu millyard. It was their first glimpse of a flying machine, and it caused almost as great a sensation as the time Nick brought the first car ashore to Kaupo—a 1916 Model T. The road in Kaupo ran only from Nick Soon's landing to his store, but Nick felt he could justify buying the car as a replacement for his mules.

Several years later, in making plans to buy a new

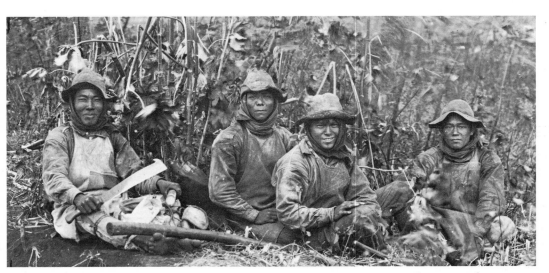

Plantation Workers

southernmost of his father's chain of stores. Nick's eight mules, sometimes each loaded with 300 pounds of rice, trod the narrow trail up from Kaupo's rocky landing. They made countless trips back and forth over the short distance to Kaupo village, which was then little more than a ranch outpost and gathering place for the Hawaiian families remaining in Kaupo, families that were among the last living in grass huts anywhere in Hawaii.

Nick later operated the family store in Kipahulu, was postmaster for Kipahulu, and was chef at his small Kipahulu coffee shop, serving chop suey, tea, and Chinese cakes.

It was with Nick Soon's help that Kipahulu would enter the twentieth century. When the first watches appeared, he learned to repair watches, and when radios came many years later, Nick became the only radio repairman within a hundred miles. He took the first photographs of Kipahulu at the turn of the century, teaching himself how to develop the film and to make prints from sepia proofing paper exposed in the sun.

The Hawaiians who gathered outside Nick's store for family portraits were surprised one day when he demon-

Model T pickup, Nick discovered that his old wood derrick was not capable of lifting the heavier new cars. No roads yet reached Kaupo, but Nick Soon was not discouraged. The maintenance of his first automobile had made him a mechanic, and he decided to build his own. He purchased all the parts he needed from eight different companies—the frame, seats, fenders, body and engine parts. He bought the bare engine block from Kahului Store and winched everything ashore at Kaupo, where he carefully assembled the parts in the backyard of the new Kaupo Store he had constructed by himself the year before. Nick enjoyed building the car so much that he later assembled a touring car and a one-ton truck.

One night not long afterward, the older Hawaiians of Kaupo were bewildered by a strange light in the Kaupo Store, a white light that did not flicker or fade during the evening. It was an electric light, the first to shine on Kaupo or Kipahulu. Nick Soon had built, from his old Ford motor, the first generator on his part of the coast.

Another of the new Hawaiians, a man who, born half a world away, would late in his life eat tea and cakes at Nick Soon's Kipahulu coffee shop, was Sentaro Ishii, a samurai.

Sentaro was almost six feet tall, unusual for a Japanese, was handsome, and carried himself proudly. In Japan he had been trained as a warrior. Disinherited by his lord, he refused to marry the daughter of the family who adopted him, and he sailed from Yokahama for adventure. A plantation recruiter had convinced him of the great opportunities in the Hawaiian cane fields at four dollars a month. He thought it was a splendid offer.

For three years he worked on Maui at Ulupalakua, then a sugar plantation. "I had never farmed in my life," Sentaro later said. "My profession was to fight with the sword." He bought his first shirt and trousers at the company store.

Sentaro learned to cook for Captain Makee, owner of Ulupalakua Plantation, and he left the field to become a domestic servant. Later Captain Clarke, part-owner of the Kipahulu Plantation, brought Sentaro with him to Kipahulu as his personal retainer and cook. Still later, when the first Japanese contract workers arrived in Kipahulu, Sentaro returned to the cane fields, this time astride a horse, his ability to speak fluently in both Hawaiian and Japanese making him an invaluable field luna.

When Clarke's partner, W. B. Starkey, became disenchanted with Hawaiian plantation life, he sold out his interest, left his Hawaiian wife Kehele, and sailed home to England. Sentaro, at the age of sixty-one, wooed and won Kehele Starkey as his bride. She owned most of the private land of Kipahulu and was twenty years his junior, although friends said Sentaro looked no older than she. He called her *Take*, the Japanese for bamboo, and named their two sons and two daughters after the plum and pine —in Japanese tradition the trees of happiness and longevity. Sentaro lived to be one hundred and two, one of the old-world men who remained to live out their lives on Hana's beautiful land.

The sugar industry prospered and the new Hawaiians continued to arrive in large numbers. Hana became a small town. The sugar company built a theater, and soon several general stores, Japanese and Chinese restaurants, and even a bakery on the main street between Ka'uiki Head and the mill.

In 1900 Hana's first hotel was established by Chinese, and in 1905 Tokutaro Okada opened a rooming house for single Japanese men. Okada shortly afterward enlarged his building to accommodate a general store that soon competed successfully with the plantation's company store. He added a soda fountain and candy counter when he married his wife Tsuru.

Ready-made clothes were not available at the turn of the century, and Mrs. Okada's pants, shirts, and raincoats found a ready market in the large number of single men on the plantation work force. Hawaiian men, resigning themselves to western clothing, became her best customers, and many Hawaiians wore their *malos* for the last time in her Hana sewing room. While the men waited for their clothes, Okada would give them a haircut for fifteen cents. By 1908 he was charging thirty-five cents, though he kept children's haircuts at a dime for many years. When he found spare time, Okada went into the forests near Hana, where he would strip bark from *ha'u* trees and carry it home to his wife, who processed it into pliable strips, dyed them bright colors, and sewed them into hula skirts for the early Honolulu tourist market.

Hana's work force grew steadily and rental rooms were in demand, so Okada added a second floor of rooms above his busy market. Okada's store quickly became a favorite overnight stop for traveling salesmen from Wailuku, famous especially for the steaming hot *furo* bath offered to guests.

Okada's store and the other privately owned Hana stores gave the company store stiff competition. Chung Kee Store, with its rows of huge glass jars filled with pickled vegetables, diverted the daily march of children on their way to the Japanese language school next to the Buddhist mission. The Ah Loon Store specialized in dry goods. There was the Takemoto Barber Shop, Nakahashi Restaurant, Kiyohiro Store, and a Portuguese bakery down the street from the telephone exchange.

Hana Plantation owned almost all the land in Hana and did its best to squeeze out the independent competition to its own store. Okada leased his land from the church, but others were unable to buy land, and most merchants leasing from the sugar company found conditions intolerable. Yet customers flocked to the private stores, which gave out gifts at Christmas, passed out candy to children and credit to anyone, credit denied workers by the company store. Because of numerous deductions, many employees did not receive any pay for eighteen months, and credit at the independent stores became very important. Japanese merchants would sometimes wait two years for payment.

Okada joined other merchants in going from door to door in the plantation camps taking grocery orders, then delivering them later on horseback. The arrangement attracted customers so successfully that the plantation manager forbade the merchants from trespassing on company property. Police were sent out to stop the deliveries.

Hana was not freed from the plantation monopoly until the death of Samuel Pupuhi, the elderly Hawaiian owner of the last privately owned *kuleana* (land parcel) on

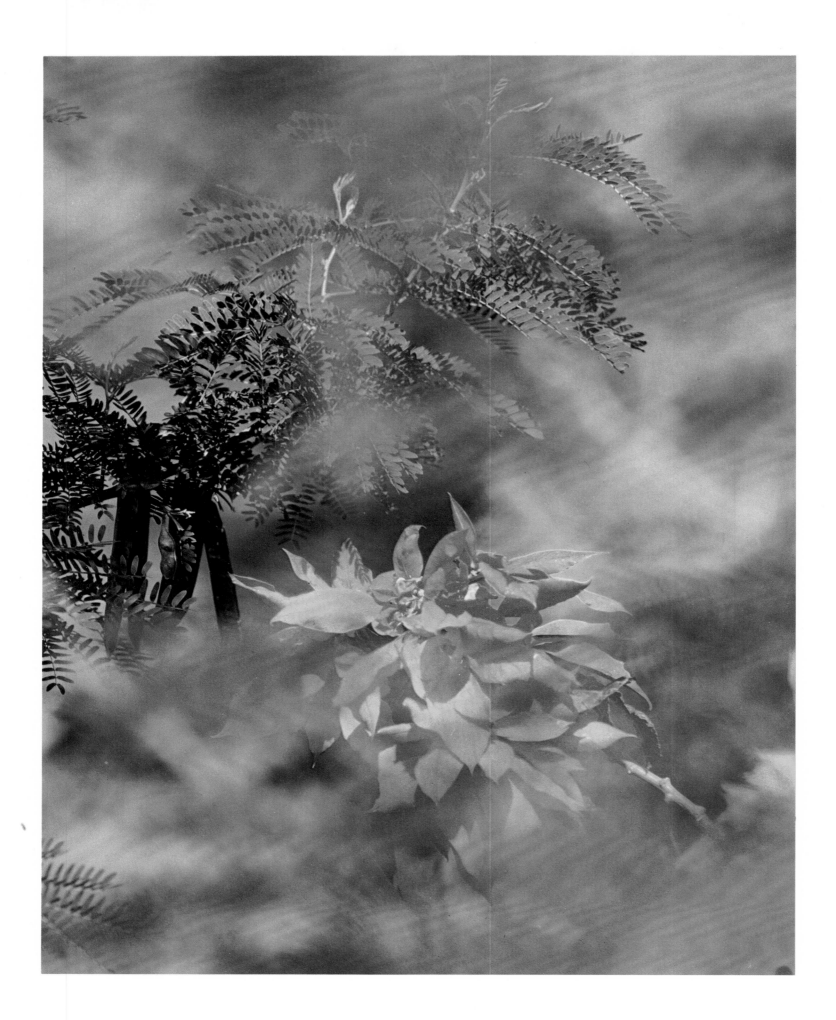

the main street. His land was divided into three parcels and purchased by Tomoji Hasegawa, who sold two of the three lots to his merchant friends. Elyno Suiso, the first Filipino merchant, constructed a store on the central lot. Kinji Kinoshita, who worked for ten years as a clerk for Hana Store, opened his own business on the parcel nearest the mill. The third lot was retained by Tomoji himself, and he opened the doors to his Hasegawa General Store in 1912.

Even the telephone came to Hana. Mutual Telephone Company's first line took thirty-two days to string through the Waikamoi and Nahiku jungles. Lines were strung across the deep gulches on poles from Oregon that were brought in by small boats and pulled by horse up the palis. The construction crew carried their own camping equipment and lived in the field. When they finally reached Hana, they found no one able to operate the exchange, and the field superintendent's family stayed on to man the small switchboard. The family handled the daytime calls, and were most accommodating to new customers, always remembering at what hours they took their baths or naps, and not disturbing them except in emergencies. Customers were equally cooperative, and refrained from making frivolous calls at late hours so as not to unnecessarily wake the superintendent, who slept by the switchboard.

As Hana grew, its social life became more varied. There were church carnivals and Japanese *Bon* dances. A second theater was built at Kaeleku, a few miles north of Hana, and Hana residents never had to worry about missing the latest movie. Kaeleku Theater played the same film as Hana Theater, but later in the evening, so it was easy to drive out to Kaeleku if you missed the first reel in Hana.

Several coastal schooners ran between Honolulu and the landings at Nuu, Kaupo, Kipahulu, Maalae, Hamoa, and the layover port of Hana. The tiny vessels were loaded offshore from whaleboats, which left Hana with sugar and molasses and returned with parts for the mills and provisions of all kinds to stock the stores.

In time, coal-burning steamers replaced the old schooners. The steamers were not required to tack across Alenuihaha Channel, and maintained a more reliable schedule. Their only delay was the early morning wait outside Hana's treacherous harbor entrance until dawn provided enough light for a safe entry.

Gliding smoothly past outrigger canoes net fishing in Hana Bay, the steamer was warped in against the concrete pier. The plantation manager from his white mansion on the hill above town could clearly hear the sounds of cargo unloading and he hurried down to check off the new mill supplies as they were unloaded. Hawaiian sailors scrambled down the gangplank in wrinkled shirts pulled quickly from sea chests, carrying ashore fish caught trolling the previous night. Impromptu parties began along the steep road into town as deckhands with a few *akule* or fresh tuna were invited in to share raw *sashimi* and Hana's famous *koji* rice swipes. The swipes were carefully prepared by Japanese field hands, the alcoholic content tested by judging the sudden whoosh made by a teaspoonful thrown over a hibachi of glowing charcoal.

The arrival of the steamer was one of Hana's great social events. The steamer would remain an important part of the Hana life—Hana's only contact with the outside world until the coming of the road.

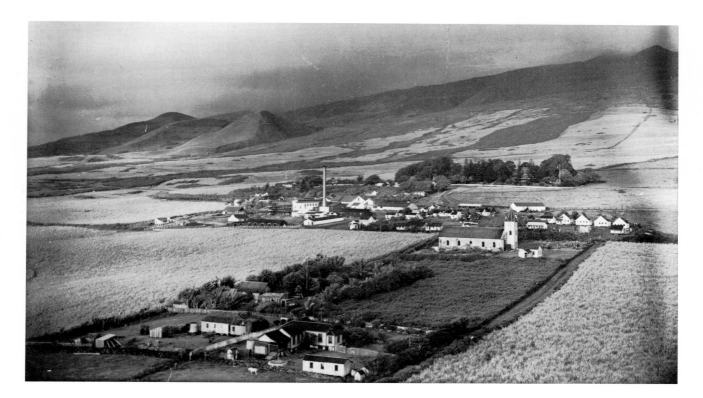

Hana, 1904

Poinsettia and haole koa, Kaupo

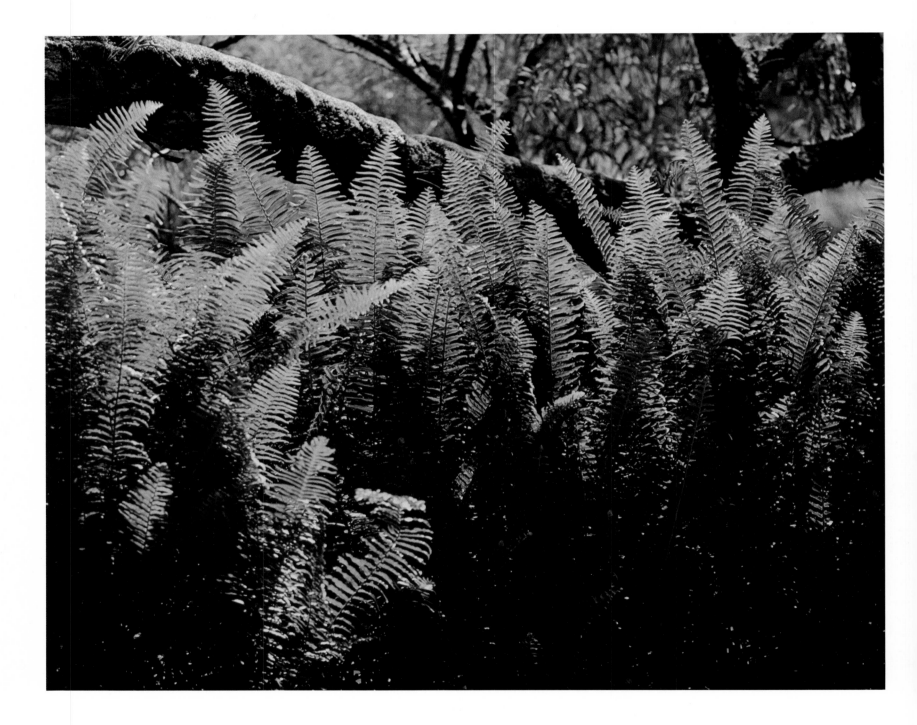

6. The Road

LONG GREEN ridges drop down from Haleakala's summit to the north shore of Maui, where at Keanae and Wailua the slope meets the ocean in a clash of black lava and blue water. A narrow road briefly interrupts this descent to the sea. The road cuts across cliffs of pandanus, bamboo, and exotic trees, and twists in and out of deep gulches. Almost every turn reveals a waterfall, and a thousand turns greet travelers negotiating the 40 miles between the cane fields of lower Paia, where the road begins, and the arid land beyond Kaupo, where the road straightens out. The roadside is a jungle of breadfruit, koa, kukui, ohia, paperbark, mango, and guava, tangled ha'u, and giant *ape* leaves, all scented with wild ginger and accented by flowers of every color.

Ha'u thickets, their blossoms slowly turning from bright yellow when they open to a deep brown when they die in the late afternoon, cover entire hillsides, making a topography of their own and shading the profusion of maidenhair ferns that grow among the cool rocks beneath. Guava trees grow together in low forests and ironwood needles fall to the ground in twos. In the spring there are red-tinged puffs of mountain-apple blossoms. In early fall, the road is covered with overripe mangoes, fallen and smashed against the asphalt. Below the road, flows of *aa* lava dip into the challenging waves, dashing aside breaking combers as if the lava were still explosively hot from Haleakala's summit.

From high roadside vantage points, there are glimpses of Keanae and Wailua villages, where Captain Cook anchored and where chiefs from Hawaii Island first in-

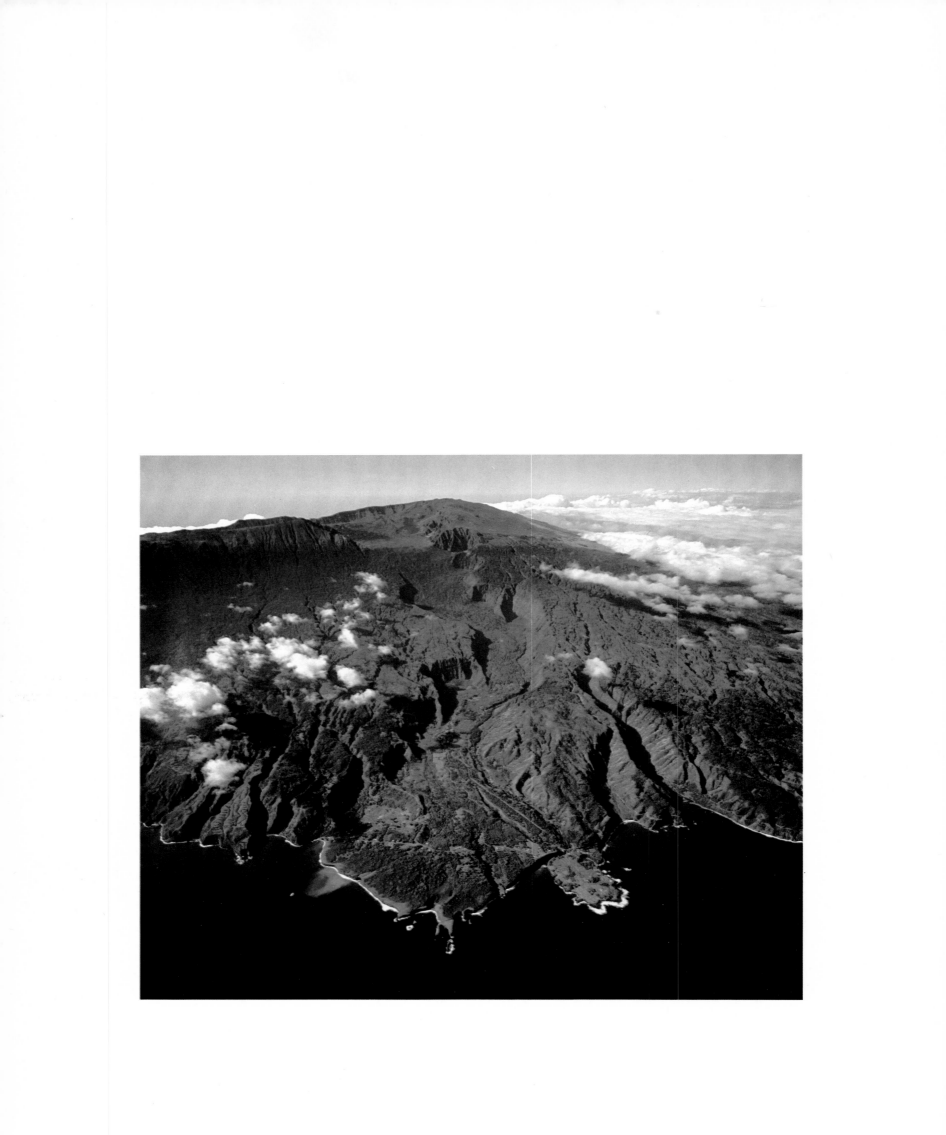

vaded the Hana district. The geometric patterns of taro patches, the coconut palms, the splayed banana leaves against weather-beaten huts, all seem images of an earlier time. Keanae village stands above the sea on a low ledge of black *pahoe-hoe* lava, and from the ledge brown villagers, sweating as warriors of another day did, launch frail skiffs and outrigger canoes across a black pebble beach into the wild surf. The last man pushes the boat free and leaps in. The helmsman pulls a knotted cotton rope and the outboard motor churns to life, the roar quickly muffled by the waves. The three men reach for their nets and prepare for a day's fishing. Ashore, the women pound taro into poi on the shaded lanais of simple homes scattered around a coral church a century old and still in use. The shingles of the houses are worn by the salt-laden winds, but the sparse interiors, protected, are highly polished island hardwood.

In nearby Wailua, St. Gabriel's mission, two bright red hearts above its entrance, stands in a neighborhood of many races, its homes neat and trim, each with a bright garden. When the builders of St. Gabriel's needed coral blocks and sand to finish construction, the waves providentially heaped the needed materials upon the shore in a single night. The residents are grateful, and the shoulders of the life-sized Christ at the cemetery gate are often draped with a lei of flowers.

Farther south along the road a miniature state park at Puakaa offers two crisp, fern-banked pools, each with a misty waterfall. Near the park, Nahiku village, almost entirely abandoned, slowly returns to the jungle. The old village landing, where coastal steamers once unloaded equipment and supplies for construction of the great irrigation ditches, is no longer used.

When Hana was without a road, and the coastal steamer arrived on a weekly schedule, Hana-bound travelers unwilling to wait for the boat drove their car to the road's end at Kailua, rode horseback to Kaumahina ridge, then walked down the switchback trail into Honomanu Valley. Friends carried them on flatbed taro trucks across the Keanae peninsula to Wailua cove. By outrigger canoe it was a short ride beyond Wailua to Nahiku landing where they could borrow a car for the rest of the involved trip to Hana. Sometimes the itinerary could be completed in a day. Bad weather could make it last a week.

Demands to extend the Kailua road to Hana were heard on Maui for years. Maui's Baldwin family were the first to request territorial money for the construction. The Baldwins, Republicans, surmised that their party would win Hawaiian votes with a modern road replacing the old Kiha-a-Piilani Highway. The family believed that the Hawaiians were ready to support any politician who did the most for them. The Baldwins were right, and for thirty-two years Republicans dominated Maui county government.

To speed up the work, a camp for Honolulu prison trustees was built at Keanae and prisoners were put to work on the road. Sections were quickly cut from the high pali extending eastward from Kailua to Keanae, but for a dozen years Koopiliula Gulch frustrated the highway builders. Not until 1926 was the road finally connected, after years of hard labor. For many months, each end of the road was in sight, separated by a slim trail across the last obdurate cliff. A great celebration in Hana followed the road's completion. Principal Haia dismissed classes for the day, and exuberant schoolchildren waving small American flags, marched down to the old cannery site on Hana Bay, where visitors driving in from central Maui joined Hana residents in a great luau that lasted for two days.

The road was little more than a wide mud and gravel path for many years until paved by a young Hawaiian contractor, Johnny Wilson, who later became Mayor of Honolulu. Even when it was paved, mudslides plagued the road. The Keanae Chinese store offered overnight rooms to stranded motorists at first, but later it became the accepted practice for drivers to wait at the mudslide for a car to appear from the opposite direction, then slosh across the intervening gap and offer to exchange cars with the complete stranger on the other side. A handshake would make the temporary trade official, and both parties would agree to meet the next day when the mud had been removed by county work crews, who usually arrived on horseback within a few hours.

The Hawaiians quickly discovered the road's merit as a fish-spotting ramp, and soon a common obstacle on narrow curves was a Hawaiian sitting quietly in his worn car, intently searching the heaving seas below for schools of akule.

Ranchers from the other side of the island also benefited by the road. The ranchers and their friends knew the land well from horseback, but the automobile offered a much easier way to treat guests to a grand tour of the Hana coast. A one-day round trip was now possible and small hotels in Hana began receiving their first tourists. The Hana road soon earned a reputation of its own—not as a road to go somewhere on, but as a destination in itself.

Keanae Valley (and the Hana Road, if you look closely)

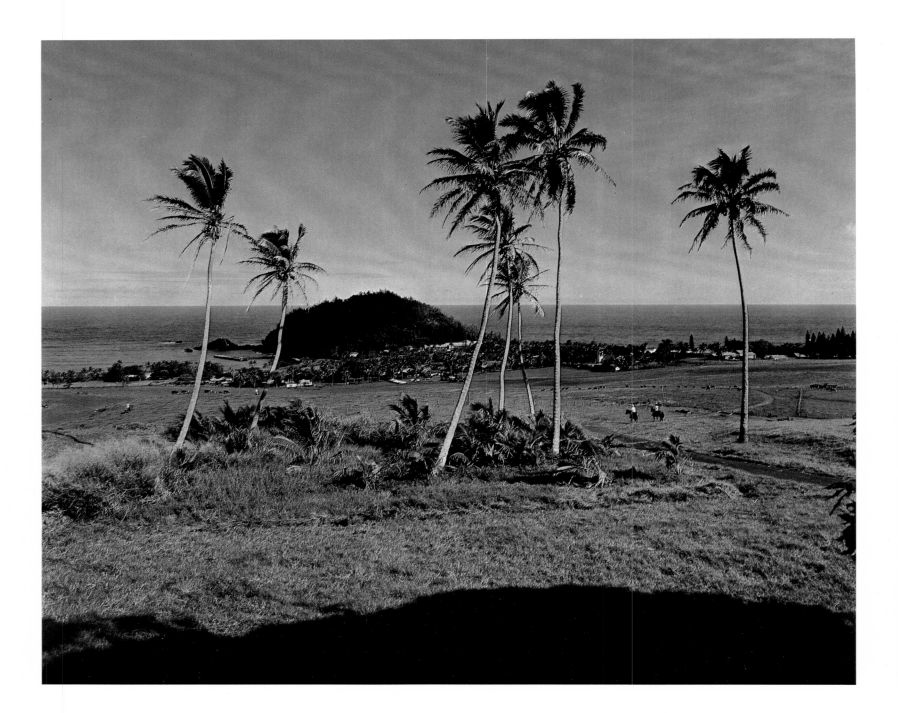

7. Cattle

IN 1940, sugar cane was growing on 1483 acres of Hana land. The Hana plantation maintained ten miles of permanent flume and twelve miles of narrow gauge railroad. It owned 44 California mules for hauling cane and 31 Hawaiian mules for hauling fertilizer. There were 4 steam locomotives, 130 cane cars, and 541 employees. The population of Hana was 1042, and it lived in 223 houses.

That was how things were when the war came to Hana. At dawn on January 28, 1942, seven weeks after Japanese warplanes struck Pearl Harbor, the U.S. Army Transport *Royal T. Frank* was torpedoed by a Japanese submarine in Alenuihaha Channel. Hawaiian fishermen on the rocks at Kipahulu saw the ship disintegrate within seconds. Survivors were picked from the oily waters by the motorship *Kalae* and taken to Hana where the plantation gymnasium was pressed into emergency use. Twenty-four islanders lost their lives.

While plantation laborers covered the Hamoa airstrip with ironwood logs to prevent enemy landings, the Army quickly established observation posts at Kaupo and atop Ka'uiki Head to watch channel waters for signs of the enemy. The local manager of the oil company wrote his head office in Honolulu for authorization to exceed the budget and camouflage the gasoline storage tanks on Hana Bay, but the next morning another Japanese submarine lobbed several cannon rounds into Maui Pineapple Company's Kahului cannery, and the manager went ahead without waiting for a reply. Sugar workers rapidly painted the huge gasoline and molasses tanks in jagged strips of grey and olive green, and the Hana sugar mill soon displayed its own proud camouflage. With this flurry of excitement, World War II passed Hana by.

Sugar was a valuable commodity throughout the war. Hana residents enjoyed a high level of prosperity that dimmed memories of past years when sugar operations barely met the payroll and the Hana plantation seemed to acquire new owners and managers with every change of the wind. Yet even during the war years, when sugar workers were frozen in their jobs, labor difficulties plagued Paul Fagan, the San Francisco capitalist who had controlled the plantation since 1930. Hana never became a popular community for bachelor caneworkers, and when job opportunities opened up in less isolated areas, the best men would leave town on the next boat.

Paul Fagan divided his time in Hawaii between Hana and a ranch on the eastern tip of Molokai where he had planned to raise prize cattle, but the old lure of Hana plantation and the East Maui coast was irresistable. He began to think of transforming the Hana sugar fields into pasture, and toward the end of World War II, when decreasing sugar prices cut into Hana's profits, he decided to buy out the other interests in the plantation, shut down the Hana mill, and establish a ranch.

The plantation's labor costs were rising, the opportunity for mechanization slim, and Fagan's partners saw a chance to be rid of Fagan, a difficult man to get along with. They allowed him to gain full ownership of the Hana plantation.

The change from sugar to cattle worked no hardship on the plantation workers. Many took the opportunity to retire. Wartime labor shortages still prevailed, and employees not needed for ranch operations were soon working for other plantations. Assistant plantation manager Ray Walker, for one, looked forward with some anticipation to a new plantation assignment. In Hana he had spent all his working hours fighting weed grass in the cane fields. Now, in 1945, he was in charge of cutting the last cane crop and—the ignominy of it!—planting grass for a ranch. The Pangola Range Grass grew marvelously in the moist Hana environment and Fagan's white-faced Herefords, shipped from Molokai, adjusted easily.

Fagan had not thought of building a tourist hotel when he first acquired the plantation, but when he realized that many Hawaiians wanted to stay in Hana, he began to think of the job opportunities a hotel might provide. The ranch could never employ more than twenty local people, and for the rest a tourist development would offer the only practical economic activity.

Tourist advisors recommended the pasture overlooking Hamoa, within a few minutes walk of the fine beach on Hana Bay. Fagan's wife Helene looked elsewhere. The

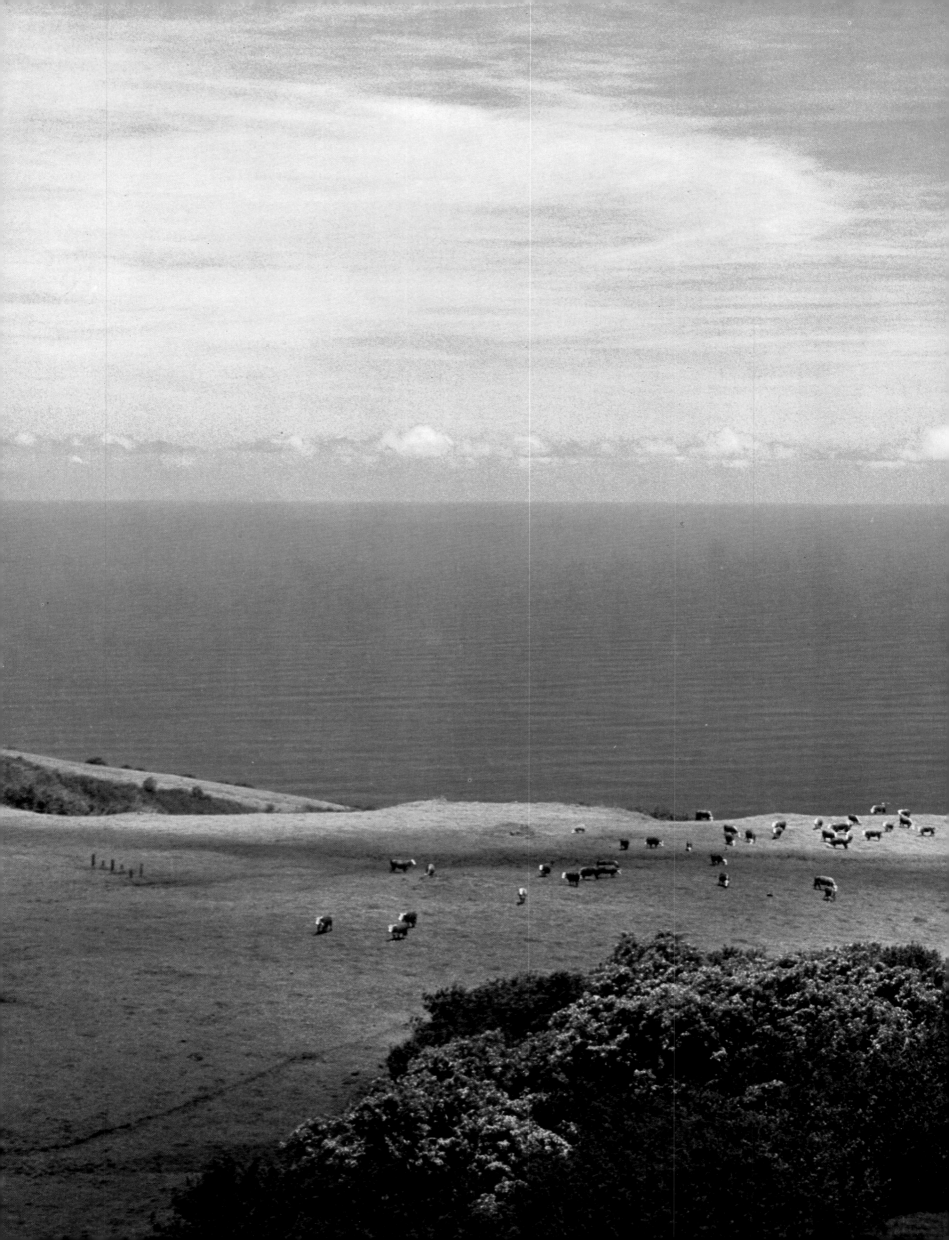

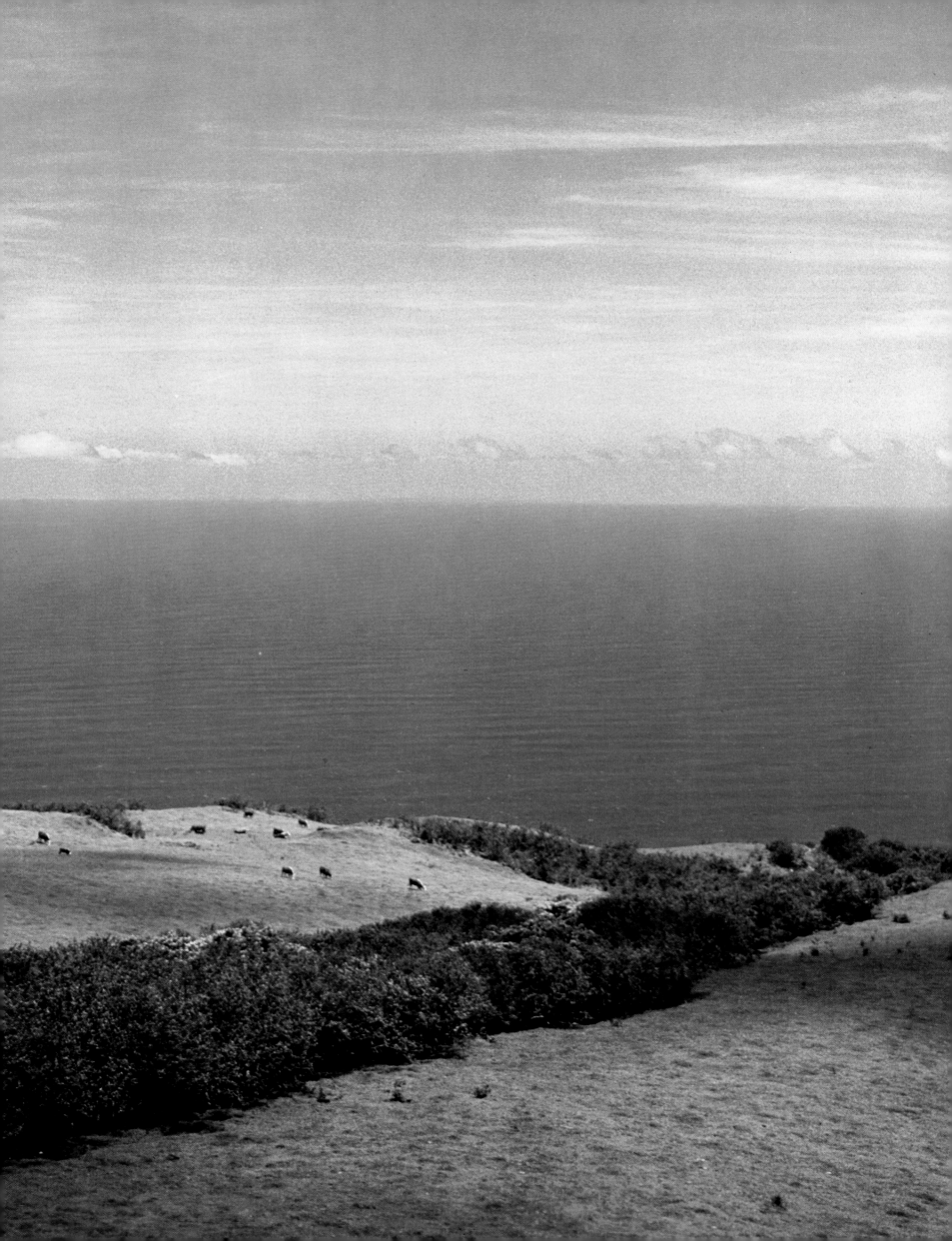

town of Hana was cooled by an ocean breeze, and she preferred it. She wanted a tropical garden around the hotel and wanted to fill the public rooms with art objects from around the world. A site well back from the sea was important, and she chose the empty block between Hana's Portuguese bakery and the old telephone exchange building, sheltered from the direct sea wind by Ka'uiki Head. They named the small hotel Kawiki Inn—Fagan's atrocious mispronunciation of Ka'uiki.

In February 1946 the first guests arrived—Fagan's own baseball team, the San Francisco Seals of the Pacific Coast League, who came to Maui for spring training. Kawiki Inn was conveniently near their practice field on the Hana school grounds. When a spring storm flooded the schoolyard, Fagan's ranch manager bulldozed a new ball park from marginal pastureland overgrown with wild sugar cane near Hamoa. It was the same field on which Kamehameha had learned to throw his spear in battle.

San Francisco sportswriters praised Hana so highly as a vacation area that Kawiki Inn was enlarged. At first the thickwalled, cool rooms designed by Fagan were occupied by wealthy acquaintances from California, who reiterated the sportswriters' claims for the place. It was said in those days that a trip to Hana was more like coming to a friend's estate than to the usual Hawaiian tourist resort. Soon, however, Fagan was dreaming of a great hotel that would combine oriental elegance and Hawaiian hospitality.

He built his hotel on the same plot of land where early Congregational missionaries had built their first grass houses, and had later replaced them with more "permanent dwellings of stone and lime, with roofs of thatch, and later of shingles." The remains of both missionary houses had long since disappeared. In 1877 the American Board of Missions, with no further use for the property, had sold the land to the Hana Plantation for $500. Not quite one hundred years later, the square block was estimated to be worth two million dollars to Hana Ranch.

April Fool's Day, 1946, dawned bright and cheerful for Hana's independent merchants, who were adjusting to the economic aftermath of the mill's closing and to the uncertainty of the future. Empty shops along the paved main street echoed new sounds—the clattering of horseshoes among others, for the Hawaiian sugar workers were turning cowboy. On that April morning, the elderly Filipino men who stayed behind rather than begin a new life elsewhere carefully groomed brightly plumed fighting birds, ruffled from a weekend of cockfighting. Japanese matrons plucked velvet vanda orchids from the *hapu* logs that stood vertically in the flower-splashed front yards of their weather-beaten plantation-camp homes.

A rolling earthquake had shaken the Aleutians earlier, but no message of warning had reached Hawaii. The long swell generated by the heaving ocean floor was then surging southward at several hundred miles an hour. Only a few Hawaiian fishermen, casting nets in shallow water at Hamoa and Keanae, saw the water receding in preparation for a great wave, and they ran excitedly seaward to gather the fish suddenly stranded and flopping wildly in rocky pools.

Few saw the enormous wave strike the unprotected shore. Some say the rolling tidal wave was thirty feet high, from its boiling foot to its high crest. The fishermen turned and ran in terror, but the great wave engulfed them. It reached shore at Keanae and Hamoa and swept inland, bending coconut palms and uprooting giant ironwoods. The sugar warehouse on Hana pier disintegrated in a solid wall of water crowding the bay. Flimsy plantation dwellings at Hamoa were smashed into pieces and their unsuspecting occupants, mothers and children and pets, were tossed about in the swirl of splintered boards and furniture.

The green mountain of water returned to the sea as quickly as it swept ashore, carrying along screaming and battered humans, cattle, and automobiles. Entire families disappeared. Others frantically clung to mango trees and the homes that remained intact. Some fled to high ground, escaping the second and third waves that swept the trim front yards clean of vanda and anthuriums. Within minutes the sea was quiet again, lapping listlessly against the disheveled shore. Friends flocked to the aid of the shattered villages, salvaging what they could, but ten houses were never found. The taro patches at Keanae were filled with a strange harvest—akule and other fish that the Alaskan wave had left behind.

The postwar years did not begin auspiciously in Hana. Hana mill closed down, then the tidal wave hit. When Paul Fagan decided to spend his retirement years there, residents could hardly guess at the future.

In the early twenties Fagan had headed a large oil company. He later pursued an importing and exporting business in Shanghai, founded and managed a Pacific Ocean freighter fleet, and owned the San Francisco Seals during the years they lost the most games. Now, as a resort hotel operator and Hawaiian cattleman, he continued to operate in his own unique way, making his own decisions and generally upsetting people, yet often finding time to be unselfish and magnanimous.

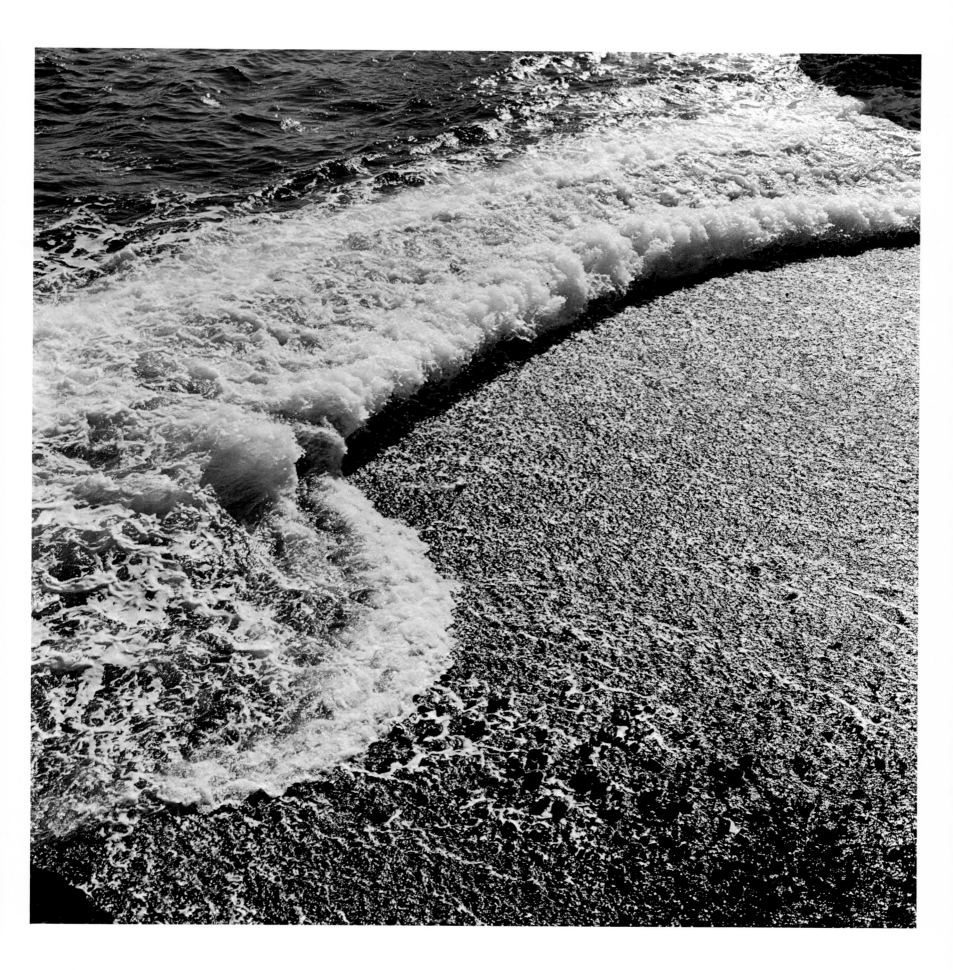

Fagan was an early riser. A 4:00 A.M. call was not uncommon. Fagan cooked his own breakfast, then met with the ranch manager to discuss the day's work. He personally inspected ranch activities on horseback, then returned before ten to change from his ranch clothes to his hotel clothes, and drive to his hotel, now the Hana-Maui, to chat with arriving tourists. He loved to escort his guests to the Hana general store and fit them with lauhala hats complete with feather leis. When the bellboys were busy he drove out to the new Hana airport to meet incoming planes, greet the visitors with flower leis and load their baggage into his car. A guided Hana tour complete with narration and a few Hawaiian words entranced the new arrivals who were lucky enough to have the hotel owner bring them to the porte-cochère. When, not knowing his identity, they gave him a fifty-cent tip, he carried their bags into the lobby.

The ranch and hotel were run in the classic paternalistic manner. Fagan abhorred unions, was convinced that he alone knew what was best for his employees, and expected them to consult with him whenever they needed help. Should they need money, however, he seldom gave a raise, preferring to explain how they might live more frugally. It was difficult to disagree, for unless one joined the county road crew, there was no other work in Hana.

Fagan's philanthropic efforts benefited Hana community and church groups on a grand scale. He organized the Hana Community Association, encouraged his wife's family foundation to grant it $11,000 yearly, and donated a $100,000 community building to Hana. A two-day luau for all Hana residents celebrated acceptance of the building, and it was named "Helene Hale" in honor of Mrs. Fagan. Fagan outfitted Hana's hospital and rebuilt the movie theater—adding a cinemascope screen and a soundproof crying room for ranch babies. He imported the Trapp Family Singers and other nationally known entertainers, paid their expenses, and opened the doors to everyone. Every man on Hana's payroll was given a day off with pay, so he could paint his own home—with Fagan paint. Every house was to be the same pale green.

When the Catholic Church decided to raise cash by selling its lands beyond Hana airport, the Church asked if Hana ranch would buy the unused grazing land for $40 an acre. Fagan, knowing the land would soon be more valuable and wishing the best for the Church, told them to wait six years. The diocese representatives duly returned in six years and asked $60. This time Fagan advised them to keep their land, explaining that its value might triple in a decade. The Church wanted cash and insisted, so Fagan paid them $100 an acre.

Individual property owners within Fagan's empire did not fare so well. Fagan was convinced that his acquisition of the Hana plantation gave him ownership of all Hana lands, especially those growing sugar cane. Many kuleana owners in Hana disagreed.

Hana's sugar industry, whose land Fagan now thought his own, had acquired much of that land by devious means. The receipts from the Hamoa Chinese store, for example, show that a free-lance land agent paid the $34.50 bill owed by a local resident in exchange for the deed to his land, nine acres that were originally part of a Great Mahele land grant. (The Great Mahele, or Great Division, was a land reform program instituted by Kamehameha IV in which Hawaiian commoners, for the first time, were given title to the land they lived on.) It was a bargain. The agent resold the acreage to Hana Plantation for a considerable profit.

Hana Plantation land agents sought out land-owning Hawaiians on other islands, offering to buy the land they had left behind in Hana. Poorly paid Hawaiians living in Honolulu quickly agreed.

In one transaction, a Hamoa Hawaiian, Kamakea, borrowed $250 from a land agent, who accepted as collateral the mortgage on the undivided interest in 22 acres. A week later, the mortgage was signed over to Reciprocity Sugar Company, which on the same day leased the land from Kamakea for fifteen years, paying him $750 after subtracting the loan. Fifteen years later, Hana Plantation, having acquired the assets of Reciprocity Sugar, transferred the leased land to their ownership records and continued harvesting cane. Neither Kamakea nor his children were notified that the lease had expired, nor that the Plantation now claimed Kamakea's land under adverse possession laws formulated by the Honolulu representatives of the sugar industry who advised the Hawaiian Kingdom.

This entirely legal procedure was repeated again and again in Hamoa, Hana, and Kaeleku. The Plantation did little to compensate the holders of undivided interests unless they complained. The few landowners who realized what was happening were paid their asking price without question.

An elderly Hamoa resident, Nalae, attempted to keep the family land untouched and undivided by creating a primitive trust. In his will, dated 1866, he wrote:

"In the name of the living God, I hereby give and devise my property unto my heirs, and to be divided as follows:

"Unto my wife, two aho (fish lines), one net, one ax, one file, one house, three hooks.

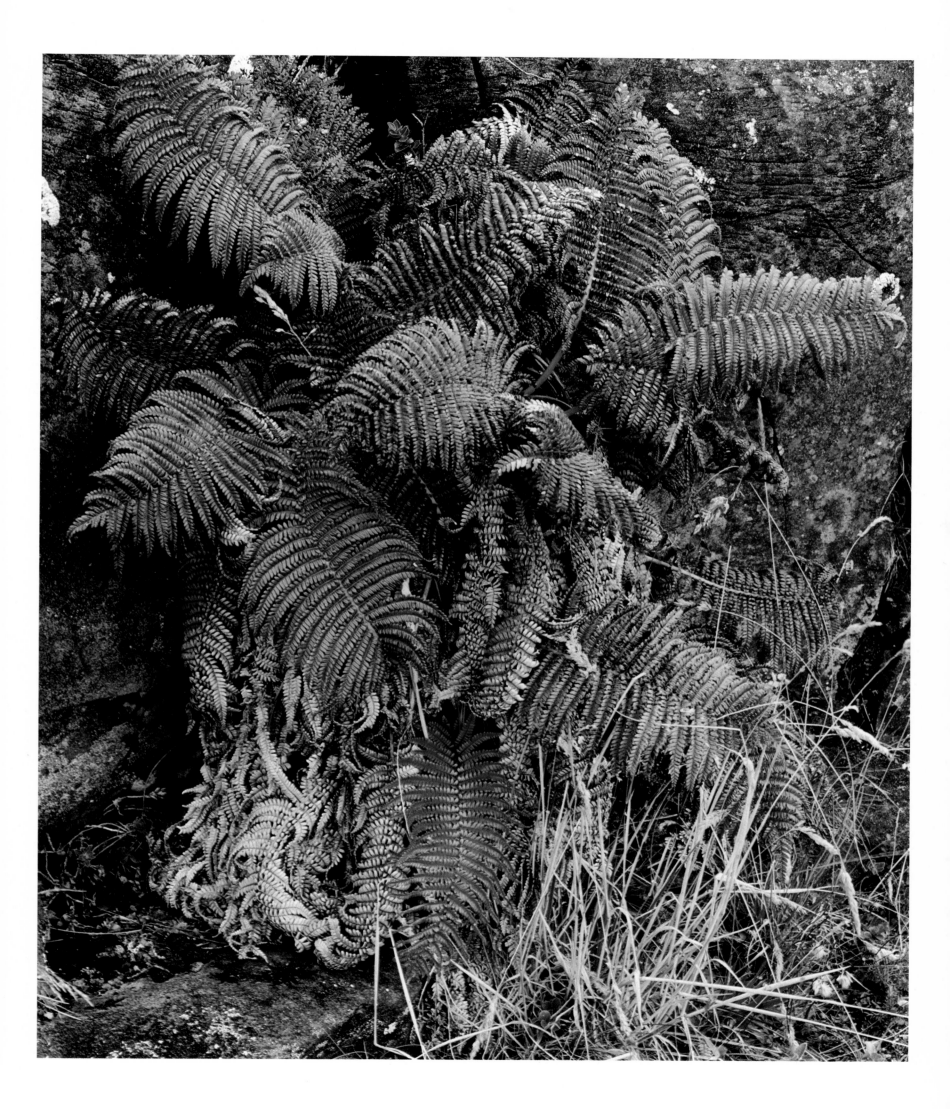

"Unto my grandchild, one aho, two nets, one large ax, one file, one package of hooks.

"Unto my son, Kamiki, I give and devise my real property, being our hui land at Mokae. This devise is for his lifetime, and upon his death he is to devise the same unto Kamila in the same manner. . . ."

Nalae's son did as the will requested, but on the son's death Kamila, who was Nalae's youngest daughter, sold one-third of the land she inherited to an enterprising Hana agent for $150. She withheld her house lot, but only until the next day, when she was persuaded to sell that too—for one dollar. The agent then sold the original acreage to Kaeleku Sugar and kept the lot himself.

Increasing numbers of children and grandchildren continued to reduce their undivided interests in the land until the fractional ownerships almost defied computation. For $75 Kaeleku Sugar purchased "not less than an undivided 315/672nd interest in and to an undivided interest in the whole land of 315/2016 in the land . . . situate at Mokae-nui . . . containing an area of 2.45 acres. The area conveyed being not less than 0.382 of an acre." The Hawaiian land ownership system had been saner than this, and Hawaiians had trouble understanding.

Older Hawaiians returned to retire on their Hana land only to find their parcels lost in a sea of tasseled sugar cane. Entire village sites were plowed under; stone walls, trees and boundary markers obliterated. The land was no longer theirs, but, by adverse possession, belonged to the sugar plantation.

Annie Pak Chong was one of the few who for years resisted encroachment by the Hana plantations, and then Hana Ranch. She gave notice to Fagan, and strung barbed wire to keep out invading ranch cattle. Annie, very much alive today, is a thin, weathered, Hawaiian-Chinese woman whose land is a remnant of a Hamoa land grant from King Kamehameha IV, now much reduced in size, subdivided and resubdivided until for the most part only fractional interests remain. Annie claims clear title and has resisted every effort to take the land away.

"When I was eight years the house was there," she says. "I remember the house was there, and my father used to raise chicken. We had a little chicken house below this on the opposite side. But I was only eight years. I'm fifty-nine, fifty-eight this year. So that's about fifty years ago."

The facts of land ownership were difficult to ascertain, and Fagan was impatient. "Why can't these people understand that I own the ranch now," he said. Fagan personally directed loading the ranch bulldozer on to a flatbed trailer, and the trailer departed for Annie's land.

"They use to rent the lands from the Hawaiians," Annie continues. "Since the plantation time, we kept on using our land because part of this was rented to the plantation and part of it, we living there. And the plantation was leasing until Mr. Fagans came here. Then he started to raise cattle and then he didn't pay us no rent for the land, no nothing. So we fenced the undivided interest and we used our interest."

In the early morning, a Hawaiian cowboy drove the ranch truck to Hamoa, towing the bright yellow D-8 bulldozer. The wide load forced oncoming cars to turn off the narrow paved road and allow the rumbling truck to pass without delay. The ranch manager, his red hair blowing in the open cab window, sat quietly beside the Hawaiian driver, with some misgivings about his morning work.

"He told us that we didn't own here," Annie says, "and I told him, I said no. I said my mother has the interest here and we own here. She lived here all her lifetime and we lived here all our lifetime after my mother. And her grandmother lived here all her lifetime. We put the fence there after the cane was over, see. So we put cattle in. He told we didn't own the place."

The D-8 was unloaded at the top of the hill. As the shiny blade bit into the wet earth covered with a stubble of grass, the machine moved forward, drowning out the sound of rocks thrown at the steel behemoth by Annie's brother. The rocks bounced off as the bulldozer easily snapped the ohia fence posts, the twisted barbed wire jerking into the air.

"He came here, he bulldozed the boundary fence. Twice he did that, on the fence we put on the boundary. We put the fence back twice. After he bulldozed it we put the fence back twice. Then afterwards, he threw me in land court, threw the whole thing in land court. It's my great grandfather's tomb that's on that round hill. It's a round tomb, on top of that hill. Yes, my mother's grandfather. And our great grandmother is over there in those trees. And my grandmother and my grandfather is buried below the beach, between the two fishpond."

Fagan's white-face Herefords slowly followed each other into Annie's green kuleana, now stripped of its boundary fence and open to grazing among the gravestones. Through years of litigation the problem of ownership of the land Annie lived on went unresolved, and goes unresolved today, but twenty years after the bulldozer felled her fence, the new owners of Hana Ranch presented Annie an exchange deed for her land. She promptly erected a new fence.

Hana pasture

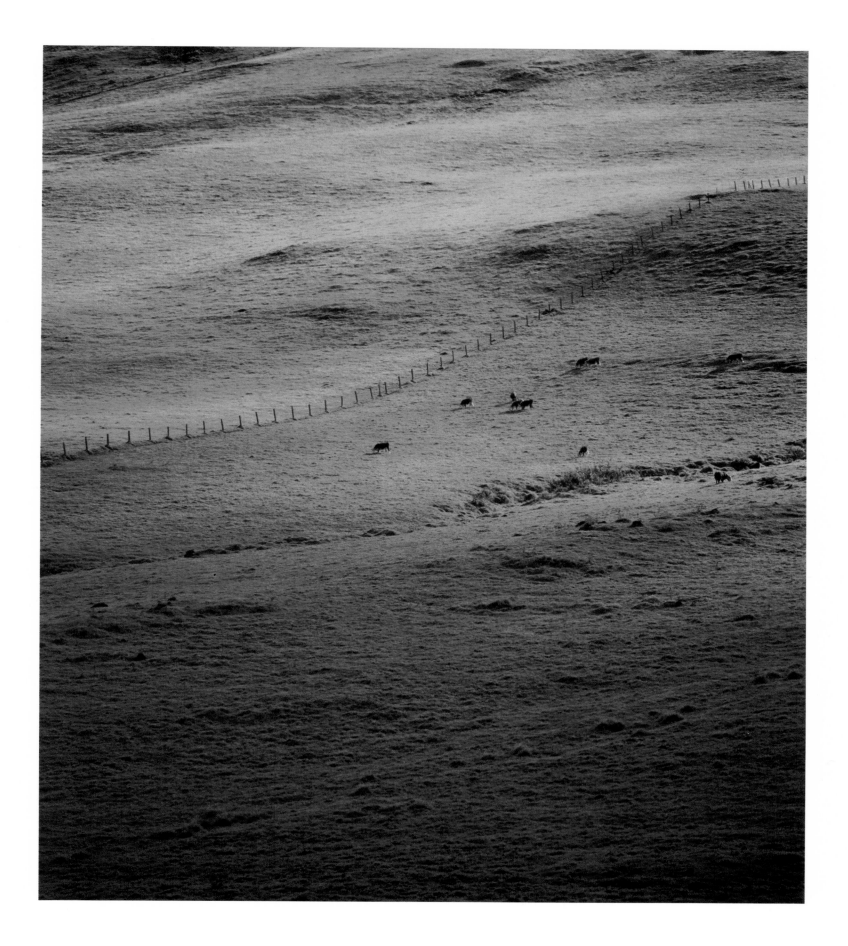

8. The Park

IN 1916, the year the National Park Service was established, President Woodrow Wilson signed into law the congressional bill submitted by Hawaii delegate Prince Jonah Kalanianaole Kuhio and thereby created Hawaii National Park. The Park included Kilauea and Mauna Loa volcanoes, and at volcanologist Thomas Jaggar's suggestion, the summit crater of Haleakala. Congress appropriated $750 for the new park.

The Haleakala section was prematurely dedicated in 1921. The first ranger-superintendent took charge seven years before all the park lands were actually deeded to the United States by the territorial government. The urgency was necessary because of increasing vandalism by thoughtless visitors who were destroying the crater's silverswords. Called *ahinahina* (gray gray) by Hawaiians, the plant is found in plentiful numbers nowhere else on earth—only on the high volcanic mountains of Haleakala. The young plants were being uprooted by visitors for the pleasure of watching them roll down the steep crater slopes like snowballs. Hundreds were destroyed by hikers who fashioned leis of silversword leaves to prove they had walked to the summit.

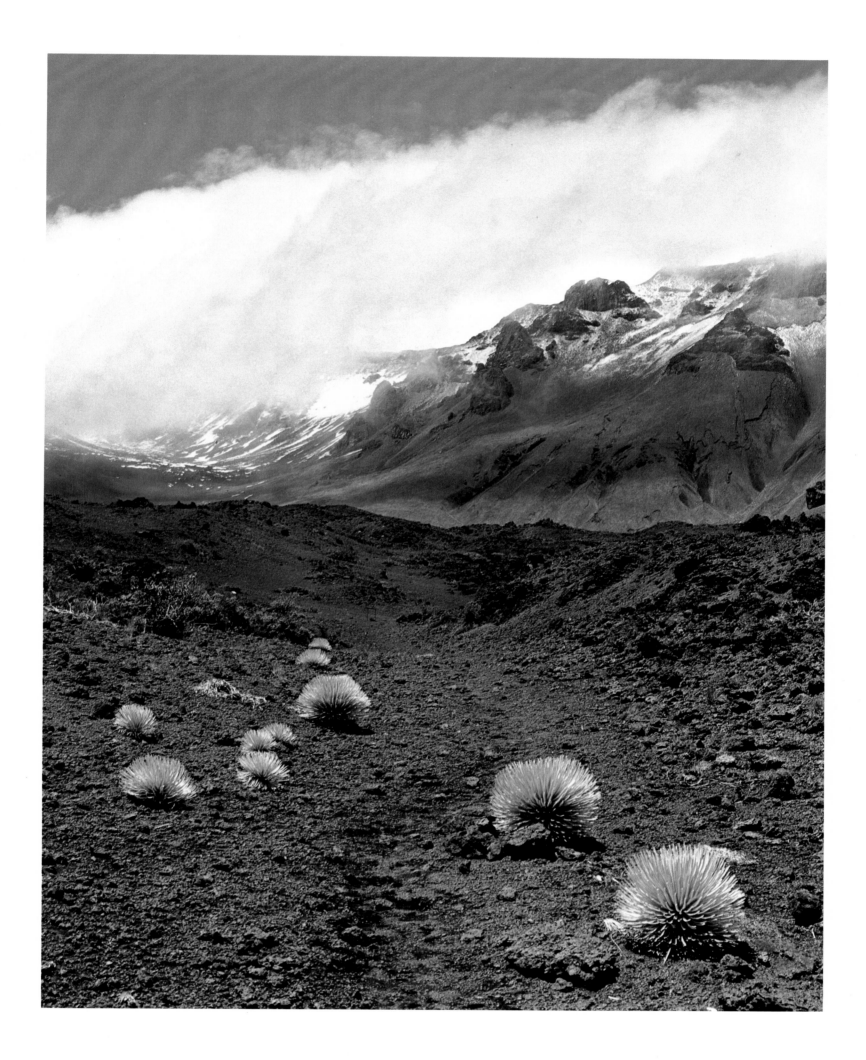

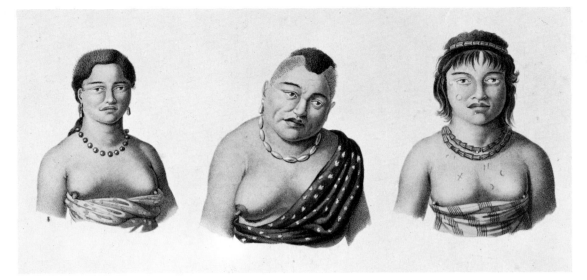

Sandwich Islanders

Local merchants were harvesting the silverswords and drying them for shipment to the Orient as decorations. Kaupo ranchers drove their cattle through the crater each summer; the cattle learned to like the tender heart of the plant and decimated silverswords along their routes of march. Feral goats ventured down from the crater rim and consumed the developing buds at will. These new enemies, in addition to the old (among them, an endemic insect that ate only silversword) were proving too much for the plant. The tall, multifoliate stalks of the silversword bloom once, then die. They produce millions of seeds, but few germinate in the crater's barrenness.

In 1929, when Otto Degener became Haleakala Park's first naturalist, he could not find a hundred silverswords. Where there were once ten-acre gardens not one plant remained. Haleakala for so long had been looked on by Maui ranchers as a combination summer grazing pasture and mountain recreation area that Park Service regulations were slow to take effect, but then silversword numbers began increasing.

There was more on Maui that deserved protection, however. A park on the Island that excluded Kipahulu and Keanae valleys was clearly incomplete. It was Kipahulu, after years of work by residents and mainlanders who knew the place, that first received consideration. The story of Kipahulu's inclusion in the National Park is a story of how the land asserted itself. The *aina alii*, the royal land of Hana, had a magic for each of the cultures that inhabited it; for the Hawaiians who named it, for the Chinese and Japanese who labored in its cane fields and

hunted herbs in its forests, for the sailors who jumped ship there, and most lately, for the wealthy men who came to build, but changed their minds.

A young Marine helicopter pilot, hedgehopping over the cinder cones deep within Haleakala Crater on a hot and windy day in 1956, was suddenly diverted from the moonscape by the frightening realization that he could not fly out over the high rim. He could only fly downward out Kaupo Gap. He did so, and shortly found himself above the Kaupo coast, with no choice but to take the long way home to the Kahului marine base, across Maui. He passed over Kaupo village and skirted the rocky shoreline in a gradual northward arc toward Kipahulu Valley.

The quiet wildness of Kipahulu was suddenly shattered by the whopping of helicopter blades. The pilot, looking down into Kipahulu for the first time, saw great waterfalls plunging from cloud-rimmed peaks and down into gorges beneath. The gorges tumbled the mountain waters to the sea at several points along the coast. Occasional, sloping fields of green along a narrow, winding road offered an infrequent white-washed building to view.

Taylor Pryor flew on in his helicopter, but the beauty that had passed below stayed with him. When the young man had left for overseas, his father had made a request, and Taylor now remembered it—that he find the most beautiful land in the world. He felt sure he had succeeded. His father, Samuel Pryor, a retired vice-president of Pan American World Airways, had set up the family's retirement criteria: beauty, good weather, water, western principles of law, and friendly neighbors. Kipahulu met the physical and legal requirements. The Hawaiian people would satisfy the requirement for hospitable neighbors.

Taylor's amateur movies of Kipahulu were screened in Samuel Pryor's Connecticut home, and the elder Pryor quickly realized that his search for a retirement home was over. He immediately called the owners of Kipahulu, one of Hawaii's great families. He wanted to buy, but the Baldwins, who owned the huge Ulupalakua Ranch of which Kipahulu was only a small part, said they never sold their land. They would gladly show him the property, however, if he wished to lease it.

Arriving for his first visit in the summer of 1959, Sam Pryor drove slowly along the rough country road at Kipahulu, marveling at the land on every side. Not in Africa, Tahiti, or Nassau had he seen anything like it. He stopped at the old sugar mill site, and looked past the broad-leafed kamani trees for the man Greg Baldwin had said would be waiting. A tall part-Hawaiian walked toward Pryor with the purposeful stride of management and introduced himself. He was William Starkey, the ranch manager and a son of Sentaro Ishii. He and Pryor climbed into a war surplus jeep and drove up the pasture.

"What do you want out here?" asked Starkey, and Pryor spoke of his retirement and how he wished to live it. They rode across the green pastures that sloped gracefully down to the sea. Across the Alenuihaha Channel they could see the hazy silhouette of Hawaii Island. Behind them rose the cliffs of Kipahulu Valley, impossibly steep

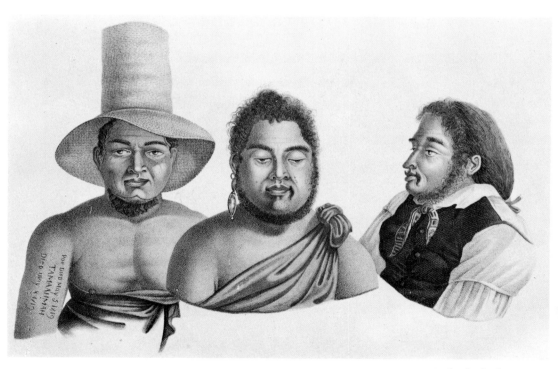

Sandwich Islanders

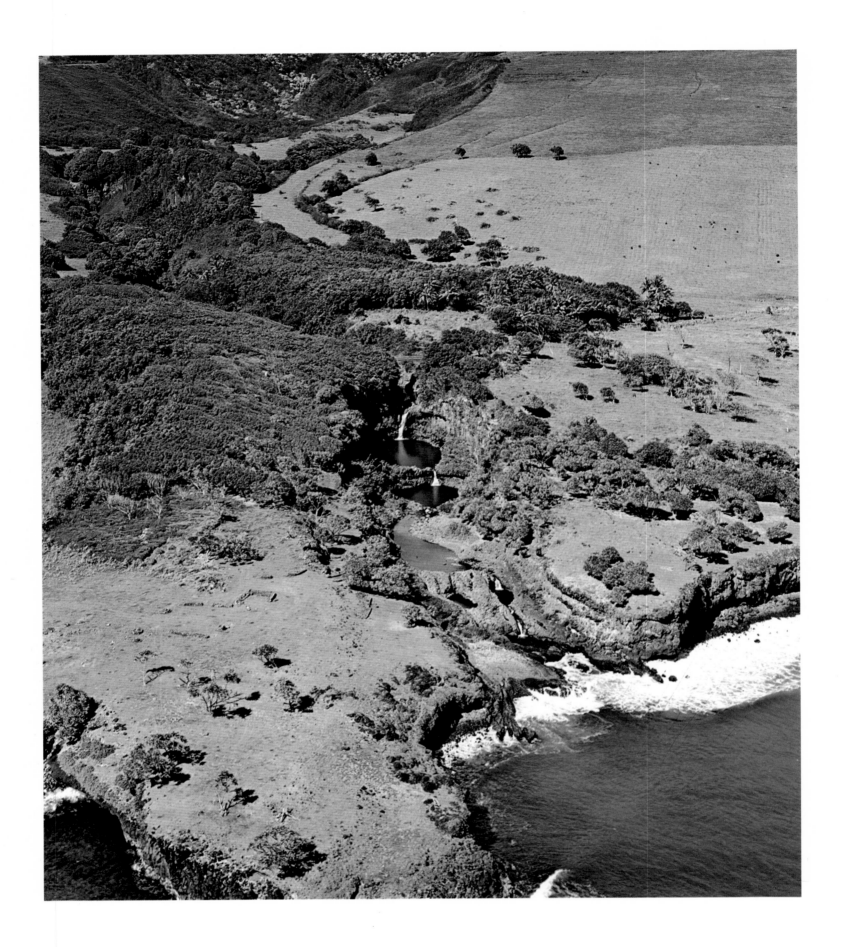

to be so green, softened with *uluhe* fern and ti. At the forest line of lower Kipahulu, the jeep stopped at the junction of two streams escaping the jungle vastness. Three waterfalls poured from high in the next valley. Everywhere Pryor could hear the sound of water. Starkey told him that Greg Baldwin, whose family owned the land, had never been here. Perhaps this is what allowed Baldwin to change his mind, for he later relented and decided to convey to Pryor one hundred acres of land anywhere in Kipahulu that Pryor wished.

Pryor camped on the land in summer and winter, sampling the sun and the rain. He finally selected a level shelf of land by Seven Pools. He chose his house site carefully. In his plans he oriented the rooms for a view of the mountains and the sea, with a short path to the lower pool where cool stream waters entered the sea down a smoothly worn lava slide. He found a clearing where he could build without disturbing the scattered pandanus trees, and welcomed the visitors who came to swim in the pools and sunbathe on the gray basalt boulders half submerged in the black sand. He told them with pride of the fine home he would build. His Honolulu architect had already completed designs for a modern, five-sided residence, with glass on all sides, inspired by the Canlis restaurant in Seattle.

Members of the Hawaiian Trail and Mountain Club, disturbed by Pryor's plans, informed him of their fears for the integrity of Seven Pools. Pryor protested, but soon realized that Seven Pools was sacred in a way he had not understood; that the simple right of public access was sacred, and that any construction would destroy the beauty and solitude of the place. He returned to Greg Baldwin and protested that he could not build at Seven Pools, because "Seven Pools belongs to everyone." Pryor exchanged the land for another parcel nearby. He crawled through the thicket of twisted hu'u trees that covered his new land, searching out the sound of water, and discovered a waterfall higher than any at Seven Pools. It was here that Pryor finally built his home.

Following Frank Baldwin's death, the executor of his estate put the entire Ulupalakua Ranch, including Kipahulu, up for sale without concern for the public interest in Seven Pools. The owners staked out a hotel site along the stream that fed the pools, placed a premium price on the land and offered the property for resort development.

It was at this time that Hamilton McCaughey, a ranch investment counselor from Reno, Nevada, born in Hawaii, flew into Hana and inspected the Kipahulu lands. He was searching for a sound ranching operation, isolated, in a beautiful setting, and was pleased to discover on his first visit that the Kipahulu lands satisfied the requirements of his client in every respect.

The Baldwin people apologized for Kipahulu Valley, saying it must be purchased as part of the larger ranch, although it "really wasn't worth it." Dick Penhallow of Hawaii's Parker Ranch recommended that he buy it. "There's isn't another ranch like it—on any island," Penhallow said.

McCaughey had first visited Seven Pools when he was eleven, traveling with his father, who as Hawaii Superintendent of Public Instruction visited Maui to inspect the Hana school and confer with William Haia, the new principal. Looking at Kipahulu from the Oheo Bridge at Seven Pools he realized that though the fields had changed from the deep green carpets of sugar cane to lighter shades of cattle range, the unique beauty of Kipahulu was untarnished. The deep, wooded valley and the gray rain showers drifting off the rim of Haleakala, still made for the beautiful land he remembered as a boy. Standing on the weathered bridge, watching the swirling water pour into the succession of pools beneath.

Two years of negotiations were required to separate Kipahulu from Ulupalakua before Jean and Ham McCaughey were able to move their temporary house trailers onto the Kipahulu lands at the site they chose to build on, not far from Pryor's new A-frame country house. At the same time, another mainland rancher, Pardee Erdman, took over the vast Ulupalakua lands in Kula and Makena.

The McCaugheys poured thousands of dollars into pasture improvements, buried jumbled piles of rock left by the plantation, and for weeks at a time assigned cowboys to plant flowering trees along the county road. Kipahulu bloomed under their care. Swimming and picnicking by local families were encouraged, and increasing numbers of tourists stopped to see the famous Seven Pools of Kipahulu, designated "the Seven *Sacred* Pools" by a hotel social director to make Kipahulu a more exciting destination.

Sam Pryor took over the restoration of Kipahulu's old Congregational church. He asked local residents about the missing pews, and one by one, each bench was anonymously returned. The ranch paniolas came by after work and on weekends to help resurface the exterior walls and reshingle the roof. He picked up an old organ in New Hampshire and shipped the aging instrument to Maui. "Boy" Von Tempsky of Kula donated a Hawaiian bible, several period church chairs were found in San Francisco, and on Sam Pryor's next trip home to Connecticut, he

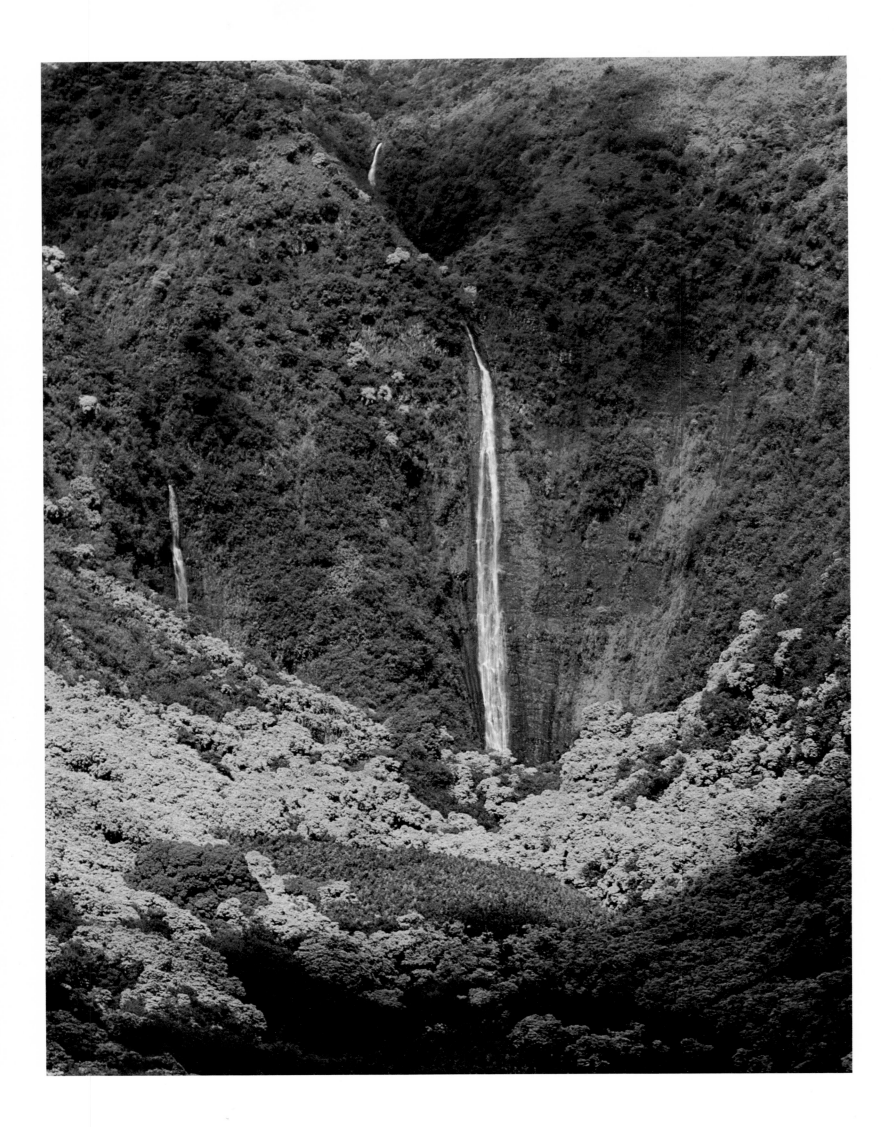

visited the same small town where the original church chandeliers were made in 1860 and he ordered a new set. On Thanksgiving Day in 1965, Pryor personally pulled the bell rope, and the old bell welcomed worshippers to the first services in twenty years.

As he came to know Kipahulu better, McCaughey became increasingly concerned with preserving its wild beauty. He watched with apprehension one day as power company survey crews began working near his ranch headquarters. Public power had not yet reached his remote land but McCaughey was convinced that the benefits of power had to be measured against scenic damage before he allowed right of entry. He conferred with Maui Electric Company engineers and they agreed to avoid clearing destructive rights-of-way through the tree-covered hillsides and to keep power lines out of sight of the winding road.

Several weeks later McCaughey's ranch employees informed him that utility crews were hacking straight paths through the jungle near Wailua. Inspection of land-entry documents revealed that nearly every easement was a line-of-sight right-of-way along the road, following the least expensive but most destructive route, contrary to the agreement he had so patiently negotiated. McCaughey and the other owners refused to sign the Kipahulu right-of-way documents. They advised the power company that Kipahulu would continue generating its own power and keep its beauty.

McGaughey and Pryor, the only outsiders living in Kipahulu, found the life fascinating. Their Hawaiian neighbors were generous, if sometimes difficult. The single twelve-party telephone line was particularly irksome. It was seldom possible to reach the outside world by phone. An important form of entertainment was playing popular records over the phone—all evening long on occasion. Romantic conversation from one gulch to the next was a popular pastime on rainy nights.

The ranch's five employees shared at least fifty children, yet even when food was scarce, the ranch workers never failed to drop off fresh akule at McCaughey's trailers or Pryor's A-frame after an early morning fishing expedition. Pryor's plans for a formal garden blossomed into a botanical extravaganza when the Hawaiians heard he was planting. They carried in everything from rare Central American pineapples to the stately Norfolk Island pine, all mixed together with every imaginable hue of bougainvillaea, ginger and plumeria. All grew well in the rich earth and Pryor's European garden was transformed into a Hawaiian backyard. The Hawaiians called everyone by their first name, and Sam and Ham quickly became the patrons of Kipahulu.

McCaughey's Kipahulu Cattle Company mailed out a brochure offering Kipahulu oceanfront property for sale, while down the road Pryor encouraged friends to build near his home, with unusual building restrictions providing that no home could be seen from any other, nor from the road. Pryor wanted them to use four-wheel-drive vehicles and drive across the pasture.

After two large parcels bordering each side of Seven Pools were sold, Annie Smith, a Hawaiian lady born at Seven Pools, approached McCaughey and reminded him of the significance of the land and expressed her concern. She liked the idea of a park embracing Seven Pools on the land granted to her family by royal decree of King Kamehameha IV during the Great Mahele. Annie Smith owned all the *mauka* pools and the best taro patches for miles around. She felt they should be in public ownership.

McCaughey called Robert Wenkam, then a State Land Use Commissioner, to ask about the State's interest. The McCaugheys were willing to sell Seven Pools at the price they originally paid for the land. Wenkam conferred with State park officials, and found that the State was not interested in making Kipahulu part of the state park system. The State saw no immediate threat to Seven Pools and gave its acquisition a low priority. Then, within the same year, the State Board of Land and Natural Resources granted special-use permits to allow residential construction on the conservation-zoned land adjacent to Seven Pools. It was clear that the State could not be trusted to guard the scenic beauty of Seven Pools, and that Kipahulu had to have federal protection.

Laurance Rockefeller had visited the Pools briefly a few years before, when Hawaii Governor William Quinn invited him to build a major resort there. Rockefeller inspected Seven Pools as a prospective hotel site, but he decided the lands were too beautiful to build upon and chose a site on Hawaii Island instead. He was informed by phone of the need to remove Seven Pools from the commercial market, and to hold the land until its transfer to public ownership as a part of Haleakala National Park. In 1967 Rockefeller purchased Seven Pools, announcing that the Seven Pools and surrounding lands represented an "outstanding conservation, cultural, and recreational opportunity . . . where the public could enjoy one of the most beautiful spectacles in the world."

Rockefeller, the McCaugheys, and Honolulu planner Walter Collins discussed buying the remaining Seven Pools land from Annie Smith, and working out an arrangement for park use of Kipahulu Ranch pastures.

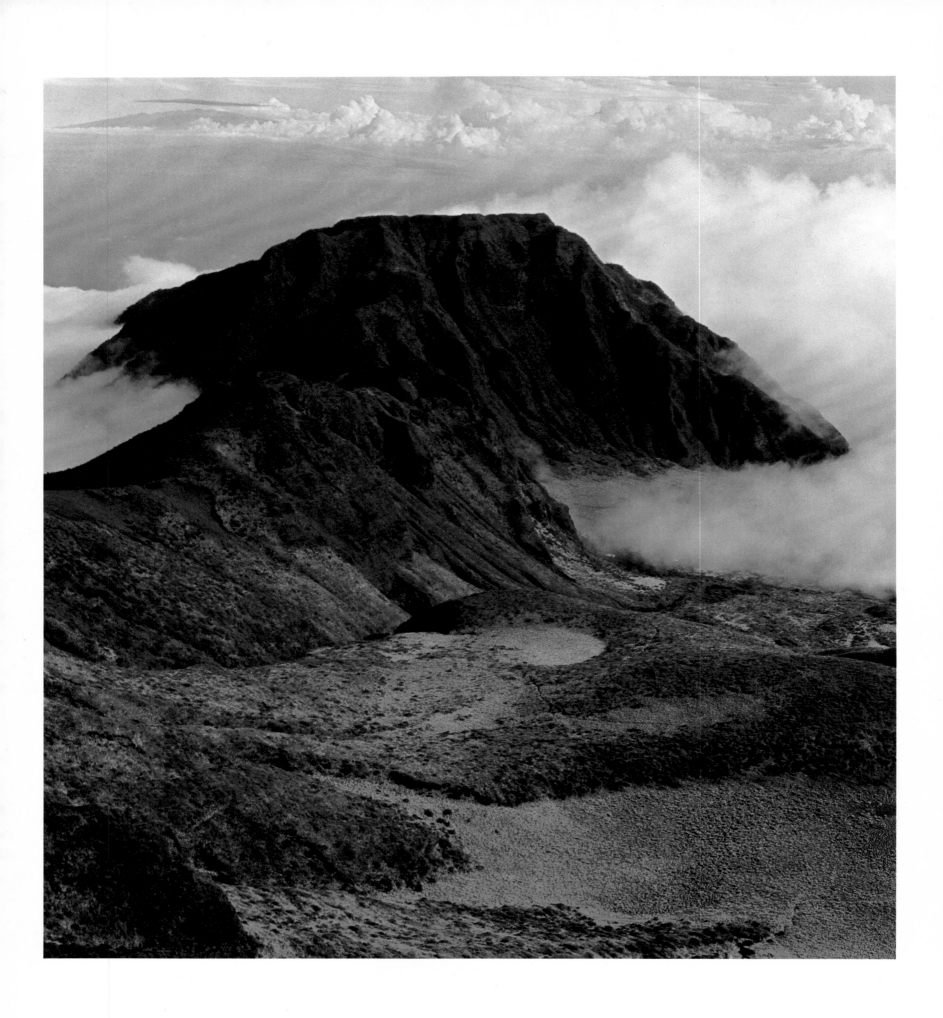

McCaughey was willing to sell 400 acres of his cattle ranch to the Nature Conservancy, and the Conservancy's regional director, Huey Johnson, was soon tramping the wet pastures of Kipahulu, evaluating their potential. He was convinced of the land's great value, and agreed to raise $415,000 in a national fund drive to buy it.

Secretary of the Interior Stewart Udall gave further impetus to inclusion of Kipahulu in the Park by reminding the Nature Conservancy that no new act of Congress was required for expansion. The act creating Hawaii National Park, now applicable to Haleakala, gave the Secretary of Interior authority to add donated lands "to round out the boundaries."

Hana physician Milton Howell and George I. Brown of Honolulu became co-chairmen of the Valley of the Seven Pools Project Committee, and within the week contributions began arriving, the first a $10,000 gift from Mary Harrison for the Mared Foundation.

Of the people involved in the fund drive, only Jack Lind, Kipahulu Cattle Company manager, had set foot inside Kipahulu Valley, and the Valley's botany was a mystery. Huey Johnson recruited a number of specialists to find out what Kipahulu held. Backed by an Interior Department grant, he organized a Kipahulu Valley Expedition to explore the remote gorge and record the rare biota that everyone assured him was there, but no one had ever seen. Jack Lind doubted that even the early Hawaiians ventured far into perpetually wet Kipahulu. His cowboys never heard of anyone's penetrating the upper rain forest. Early records tell of a few scientists who did penetrate. They were bird collectors, and they found the going rough. An 1892 diary relates that the valley was extremely wet: "When we pitched the tent today we had the greatest difficulty to fix the poles, so soft and swampy was the ground, and torrents of water were running down the slopes . . . and we never had so much difficulty in making up our fire. The forest here has a wild and peculiar aspect, dead fallen trees lying everywhere in one's way and others standing lifeless and leafless between the green ones."

In 1945 three park rangers nearly lost their lives struggling without guides through the Kipahulu rain forest from the rim of Haleakala, and over the years others have reported making the strenuous trip, but not until the Nature Conservancy launched its well equipped expedition, with time to devote to basic research, were Kipahulu's secrets revealed.

The expedition started out on the second of August in a torrential rainstorm and twenty-eight days later emerged dripping from the jungle. It was still raining. At the base camp the ranch hands aiding the expedition logged huge hapu tree ferns and laid them side by side to make dry platforms above the deep mud. Fern fronds piled on top of the irregular surface made a mountain mattress on which tents were pitched and equipment secured. One night during the first week it rained nine inches, leaving the scientists stranded in a sea of brown water. The inundation almost ended the expedition, but the scientists stuck it out, and went on to compile the first record of what proved to be a wilderness of great ecological importance.

Expedition leader Dr. Richard E. Warner in the Kipahulu Valley expedition report writes that "Kipahulu Valley is, without a doubt, one of the outstanding areas of the Hawaiian Islands for native birds. The opportunities for research in this unspoiled area are legion." He reported the sighting of a Maui *nukupuu*, previously considered to be extinct, and three other species on the International Endangered Species List.

Expedition member Dr. Charles Lamoureux wrote, "We have recorded about 220 species of higher plants in the valley. Of these only 10 per cent are species introduced to Hawaii by man. . . . Since most of the Hawaiian species of plants are endemic, these communities are like no others, and Kipahulu in this sense offers an opportunity not available elsewhere on this planet."

"Looked up the valley—had to be something up there," Huey Johnson had remarked of his first walk in Kipahulu. The expedition had confirmed his intuition. On October 14, 1968, a year after the expedition tramped bedraggled out of Kipahulu, a Conservancy-sponsored reception in New York City raised more than $221,000 and large grants in following weeks sent the fund drive over the top. Johnson gave most of the credit to Warner's expedition and the indefatigable services of Dr. Milton Howell, Hana's country doctor, who bounced contributors across the Kipahulu landscape in a Land Rover between stints at the small local hospital where he is the only doctor within the seventy-five-mile length of the district.

In the final negotiations the Nature Conservancy purchased the privately owned half of Kipahulu Valley and received as a gift 400 acres of lower ranch pasture from Jean and Hamilton McCaughey and 52 acres at Seven Pools from Laurence Rockefeller. Although at least 500 acres more would have to be purchased to assure the integrity of Seven Pools (and have yet to be purchased), it was decided immediately to conclude transfer of the lands to the National Park Service under the Johnson administration, and on January 10, 1969, Secretary Stewart Udall signed the documents extending Haleakala National Park from the summit rim to Kipahulu's coast.

9. A Proposal

THE SIMPLE enlargement of Haleakala National Park will not be enough to preserve East Maui's uniqueness, its spirit of place. Much of what is unusual about the Hana coast lies outside present or proposed park boundaries, and is vulnerable. The bit of old Hawaiian life that is lived in Kipahulu, Keanae, and elsewhere on East Maui needs the same protection as the wild birds of Kipahulu and the silverswords of Haleakala receive from the National Park. A conventional park cannot supply that kind of protection. Clearly, a new concept in environmental preservation will be necessary for East Maui. Its concern must be for the total environment; for the land, wildlife, and culture of a piece of island. [*See map facing page 160.*]

To this end, Friends of the Earth and the author propose a complex of one federal and several state and county parks, linked by a simple parkway, with park boundaries protected by zoning regulations and scenic easements, and limitation of park visitors if their numbers become overwhelming. The plan will require imagination on the part of the National Park Service and cooperation between federal, state, and county agencies. It will require the same farsightedness on the part of Maui landowners that they have shown in the past. It will take considerable hard work and thought, but will be the best way of assuring that future generations know what the good land and life of Hawaii was like.

THE NATIONAL PARK. At the heart of the proposal is an enlarged Haleakala National Park. This larger park should have the boundaries that the old Hawaiians would have given it, for in their centuries on the land the native people evolved a sensible system of managing it. We would be foolish to ignore the native expertise.

The early Hawaiian chiefs divided the Maui land into slender, pie-shaped parcels called *ahupuaa* that extended from the summit to the sea. Each chief thus had a bit of slope and a bit of shore. He and his people could satisfy all wants from the produce of their own land: shellfish, beachstones for building, and taro from the coast; pigs, logs, and feathers for alii capes from the higher forest.

Haleakala Park should extend, like a large ahupuaa, from the summit to the sea. The Park does almost meet the sea at Seven Pools, with the recent Kipahulu Valley addition, but Kipahulu is only one leg, and it reaches only tentatively toward the water. Haleakala Park needs another leg to the sea—at Keanae—and its Kipahulu section needs enlargement. With these two good legs, Haleakala National Park will stand complete. It will include all the life zones from two sides of the island, and will contain within its borders a number of Hawaiians following each of the ways of life that Maui's history has known, with the exception of the sugar plantation life (and there are old mill ruins and plantation churches to give Park visitors an idea of that).

The park should also be expanded to include the grasslands above Paliku, Manawainui Valley, and a buffer zone downslope from the crater rim.

KIPAHULU. Kipahulu Valley is perhaps the last true wilderness in all Hawaii. Kipahulu's native forest is almost completely free of the introduced plants and animals that are well established everywhere else in the Islands. Feral pigs do climb the valley walls and a few foreign flowers do grow among the mixed roots of koa, fern, and lobelia of the valley's swampy floor, but otherwise the valley remains as it was before the first Polynesian voyagers arrived at Kahikinui, a few miles away.

Botanist Charles Lamoureux of Hawaii describes Kipahulu Valley as an area of "unequaled opportunity to preserve an entire, unique ecosystem almost undisturbed by man and his activities." Lobelias unique to the valley, and numerous rare grasses and ferns grow safely there. The tangled trunks of ohia lehua, bearded with moss and enshrouded commonly by fog and rain, shelter the last of Maui's hook-billed nukupuu, until 1967 thought to be extinct. The rare Maui parrotbill, the crested honey-creeper, and the Maui creeper—all endangered species—survive only in the ohia forest of Kipahulu Valley.

This Kipahulu jungle, though vast and wild, is vulnerable, its ecology delicate, and man must step gently here. The park boundary must be expanded to include lands beyond the narrow ridges that enclose the valley, in order to accommodate a trail from the summit to the sea, a trail that will not scar the palis of the valley walls, or intrude on the valley floor. A hard-surfaced trail within the valley would disrupt the fragile ecology of Kipahulu's bog. Exotic seedlings would inevitably spring up along its length, and pack animals would bring down its giant koas, for hoofs are not compatible with shallow root systems.

The highlands above Kipahulu also should be included in the park. At 9000 feet, a tabletop landscape of native bunchgrass protects the head of the valley, but in addition is worthy in its own right of inclusion in the park. This high country is where Maui's weather is born; where warm winds, rising up Haleakala's slopes, meet the tropical inversion layer and fall back as rain. Here, sheltered by narrow ridges and seldom seen, are the tiny lakes Waianapanapa and Wailele'ele.

The lower, pastoral country of Kipahulu, though perhaps not as vital to the park as the wild country above, should nevertheless be an integral part of the park. Below the edge of Kipahulu's forest, the gently sloping land has been planted in sugar cane or grazed by cattle for more than one hundred years, and bears little resemblance to the pristine land it was when its marginal taro patches were fought over by warring chiefs, and its darker depths hunted by canoe builders and feather collectors, superstitious men who started at strange noises, imagining the *Menehune, Mu, Akua,* and other supernatural tribes that lurked out of sight. Twentieth-century man's mark here has been deliberate but kind. The simplicity of the pasture contrasts strongly but pleasingly with the profusion of the forest above.

Kipahulu's pasture will never be wild forest again. When the cattle cease to graze here, impenetrable groves of Hawaiian Christmas berry and guava begin to grow. The guava and lantana, thickets of blackberries, and other aggressive plants are all contents of a Pandora's box of alien vegetation, brought to Maui by plantation owners and traveling botanists, a box that once opened gave native plants no chance. The cattle, then, should continue to graze in lower Kipahulu. The pastures should remain part of a working cattle ranch—a bit of living history—under a concession arrangement with the National Park Service.

KEANAE. The lava peninsulas of Keanae and Wailua, their black basalt foundations long since softened by green growth and human habitation, are peninsulas out of time. With a few concessions to this century, like the outboard

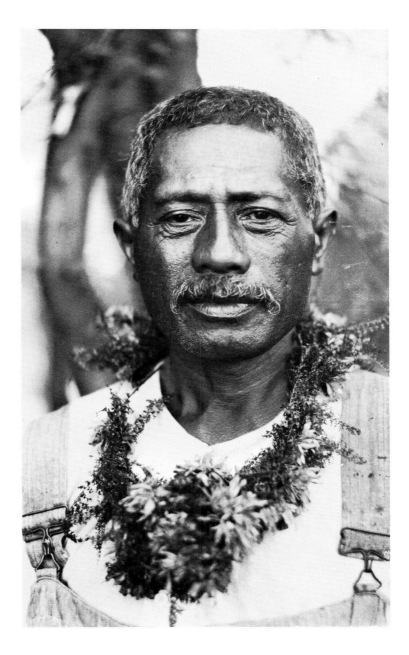

Kaliko Makakoa, Hana

motor, the people here live an old Hawaiian life. They grow taro and they fish the coastline as their ancestors did. The same green geometry of taro field that greets visitors today greeted Captain Cook.

The National Park must not disrupt the traditional land-use patterns of the peninsulas. (The park, in fact, may be the only way to preserve those patterns. However healthy and satisfied the Keanae community appears today, urbanization marches on and pressure for change mounts.) The kuleanas of resident families, held since the Great Mahele of Kamehameha IV, should become provinces within the park. Tax incentives, perhaps even outright subsidy, should be employed if for any reason— a failure of the taro market perhaps—the peninsula residents need encouragement to remain on the land.

At Cades Cove in Tennessee's Great Smoky Mountains National Park, the pioneer way of life is preserved as an integral part of the park much as Keanae, Wailua, and Kipahulu might be preserved in Hawaii. John D. Rockefeller, Jr. purchased most of the land at Cades Cove and donated the parcels to the National Park Service. Descendants of the original farmers were given first rights to lease back the land under agreement that the land be maintained in its condition at time of settlement. The residents pay no land taxes because the farms are government owned. The lease agreement, with an option to renew, calls for a rent payment to the government of only one dollar per acre per year, allowing for programs of improved farming practice, better livestock, and, when necessary, new homes built in the pioneer architectural style. Inclusion of Maui's taro-growing peninsulas within Haleakala National Park under such lease-back agreements may be their only choice for survival.

The Keanae life is important because it is different, and diversity is the commodity that is leaving the world fastest. Even on East Maui, great sugar cane, pineapple, and range-grass monocultures have replaced with their uniform greens much of the complexity of the native ecosystem. And one trouble with monocultures is that they are monotonous. Plant cultures, and human ones, need variety if they are to be interesting, and stable. The life in Kipahulu and Keanae is a variation. It's not Honolulu or Hilo. The approach to life is calmer, and different. The spirit here is Hawaiian, even when the clothes and old sedans are not. In including Kipahulu and Keanae in the National Park, we will have more, then, than dead historical displays in a visitor reception center, more even than a living museum; we will have salvaged some of the planet's vitality.

THE STATE PARKS. East Maui at present has a number of state parks, most of them roadside miniparks created at stream crossings by the State Division of Forestry. It's a good terrain for tiny parks, and some of them are exquisite, but they are too small to provide real protection for the country along the Hana road. The groves of marketable Eucalyptus robusta and native acacia that shade the road will soon need the protection of better parks.

Most of the existing parks are surrounded by extensive state-owned acreage, and park enlargement could be accomplished simply, without cost, by executive order of the governor. State park status, without improvements of any kind, will give assurance that many miles of roadside forest will not be endangered by unwise grazing leases or timber sales.

East Maui is a countryside where beauty is a common roadside commodity, often taken for granted by citizens whose backyards would qualify for park selection if study teams looked in on them. Certain places do stand out, however. The pandanus forests at Waianapanapa and Ulaino, the redwood and cypress covered slopes of Poli Poli Springs, and the slender waterfalls pouring from the hills above Wailua Valley all deserve state-park status.

THE COUNTY PARKS. The recreation needs of the Hana community, and the needs of visitors who come for water sports, can be served appropriately in small county beach parks at Honomanu, Hana, Hamoa, and Nuu bays, all easily accessible from the highway and nearby towns. The surf of Keanini along the north of Hana Bay and the pebble beach at Wailua, from which canoes were launched in the old days, should both become county parks, protected from a private development demeaning of their historical significance and incompatible with their public use. County and state park boundaries might also be extended beyond the shoreline to include the surf and underwater country beneath.

An improved system of state and county parks, by involving local authorities in the responsibility for Maui's environmental integrity, will give the conservation effort on Maui a political strength it could not otherwise have. But more important, state and county parks will relieve pressures on the national park. The subordinate parks will accommodate those who come for automobile camping, for land sports like baseball and tennis, and for the activities associated with the sea—surfing, fishing, boating, gazing. The national park itself must never become an overnight recreation area. Haleakala Park's purpose must always be that described in the National Park Act—the use of natural features by such means as will leave them unimpaired for the enjoyment of present and future generations. Recreation in Haleakala should remain limited to the outdoor experience of those willing to walk to a distant cabin. And some places should be known only by what they tell the eye and the ear and by the aromas that come from a distance.

For additional protection against development within

the park, visitor centers could be established at the Huelo, Hana, and Kaupo entrances to the park. The centers would provide low-cost hotel and motel accommodations to supplement the higher priced hotel and cottage accommodations already present in Hana, and those that may be built there, thereby satisfactorily filling the needs of park visitors of every degree of affluence.

A STATE WILDERNESS. The upland jungle of Nahiku, an outstanding wilderness study area because of its relatively undamaged condition and its considerable size (fifty square miles) should become a wilderness preserve. Nakihu needs preservation. The National Academy of Sciences lists the Maui biota as "among the most critical in the world because of their exceptionally high endemism and the rapidity with which they are disappearing before the onslaught of man and introduced species of plants and animals." The high endemism makes Maui a natural laboratory for the study of evolutionary processes. Hawaii's long-horned beetles, of which there are 6 genera and 110 or more species, are, according to the Academy, an outstanding example of how insularity allows for dramatic evolutionary radiation. Maui's rare land snails, its honeycreeper, and all its other unique species should be protected for future study. The Nahiku Wilderness would provide the study area.

THE PARKWAY. East Maui already has a parkway, though it is yet to be dedicated. The Hana road is already one of the world's great scenic drives. It would be impossible to improve upon the road; higher engineering standards would be disastrous. The road now meanders, crosses narrow bridges, and is littered often by fallen mangoes, but there is nothing wrong with that. The mangoes are still good to eat. The grass grows to the edge of the road, and mongooses run from its cover to disappear in the grass at the other side. If the road were wider and faster, mongooses wouldn't make it. Today they have plenty of time, but if East Maui's future holds a freeway, mongooses will have to take their chances, as the jackrabbits of the western states do. The road should be left alone. Fallen mangoes are a more acceptable litter than fallen mongooses.

The view from the parkway should be protected by scenic easements, the common practice with parkways. There are special problems on Maui, however, and the parkway, like any feature of an environmental master plan, would require innovation.

The Blue Ridge National Parkway in the Shenandoah Mountains of Virginia is closest to what the Hana park-

way might be, but unlike the Blue Ridge Parkway, the Hana parkway will have no back roads to carry our farm produce or supply the communities along its route. The construction of such roads would be enormously expensive and enormously destructive to the terrain. All traffic, therefore, must use the single road. Fortunately, Hana's commercial traffic is sparse. An occasional taro truck on a working road that is part of a living community, will not be a bad thing. If heavy trucks on the narrow road should prove a problem, more freight could be routed to Hana's airport. Already Hana beef is flown on the hoof to Honolulu. The often quiet airport could easily handle more business.

The Hana parkway will not be a road to get somewhere on—it will be its own destination. The airplane to Hana will carry the impatient.

ENVIROMENTAL ZONING. The inevitable attempts at commercial exploitation of national park boundaries by souvenir salesmen and motel operators may be controlled through federal acquisition of development rights for land adjacent to the boundaries. We can predict that many residents will act to protect the integrity of their neighborhoods by donating development rights to tax-deductible landholding trusts like the Nature Conservancy.

Maui County in its turn could strengthen the environmental master plan for East Maui by acquiring line-of-sight scenic easements to protect the County's scenic views. Cooperating landowners would receive the tax benefits due them under Hawaii's state land-use law. (Landowners would also benefit in that the value of property almost always increases when a national park is dedicated near it.)

The Hana coast should never be burdened by a mountain freeway or speculative subdivision or high-rise hotel. Maui's primary tourist destination areas must remain on the western side of the island. A look at the map will show that this western concentration of resorts has been the pattern of the past. It would be admirably sensible if Maui, through zoning ordinances, kept it as the pattern of the future.

HANA TOWN. The new owners of Hana Ranch have dedicated themselves to a policy of land management designed to preserve the Hana environment. The Ranch shareholder's profit in Hana will be limited by environmental considerations. Determining an optimum tourist population and an optimum resident population will be the primary concern of the Ranch master plan. Ranch President Tap Pryor and the Ranch owners are convinced

SOURCES

ADLER, JACOB. *Claus Spreckels, the Sugar King in Hawaii.* Honolulu: University of Hawaii Press, 1966.

ALLEN, GWENFREAD. *Hawaii's War Years.* Honolulu: University of Hawaii Press, 1950.

AMERICAN BOARD OF MISSIONS. *First Ten Annual Reports of the American Board of Missions for Foreign Missions.* Boston, 1834.

APPLE, RUSSELL ANDERSON. "A History of the Land Acquisition for Hawaii National Park." Unpublished thesis, University of Hawaii, 1954.

ASHDOWN, INEZ M. "Maui History." Unpublished notes, Maui Public Library, 1951.

BALDWIN, ARTHUR D. *Henry Perrine Baldwin.* Privately printed, 1915.

BARBER, JOSEPH, JR. *Hawaii: Restless Rampart.* New York: Bobbs-Merrill Co., 1941.

BARTHOLOMEW, HARLAND, and Associates. "Economic Evaluation of the Proposed Keanae Extension, Haleakala National Park." Prepared for the U.S. National Park Service. Honolulu, 1964.

BEAGLEHOLE, J. C. (ed.). *Journals of Captain James Cook.* Cambridge: Cambridge University Press (for the Hakluyt Society), 1967.

BELL, A. D. "The Hawaiian Slavery Slander" (editorial), *The San Francisco Merchant* (San Francisco), January 26, 1883.

BINGHAM, HIRAM. *A Residence of Twenty-one Years in the Sandwich Islands.* Hartford: H. Huntington, 1847.

BRADLEY, HAROLD WHITMAN. *The American Frontier in Hawaii.* Stanford: Standford University Press, 1942.

BROWN, A. B. "Trail Blazing on Maui." Unpublished manuscript in Maui Public Library, Waiakoa, Maui, Hawaii.

BROWNE, G. WALDO. *The Far East and the New America.* (Includes article on Hawaii by Senator Henry Cabot Lodge.) New York: The R. H. Whitten Co., 1901.

BUDAR, VALJEANNE. *Paul I. Fagan, Baron of Hana, Maui.* Honolulu: Paradise of the Pacific, 1957.

"C. Ah Ping Recalls Days when Molokai grew Sugar Crops," *Honolulu Star-Bulletin,* September 8, 1939.

CHEEVER, HENRY T. *Life in the Sandwich Islands.* New York: A. S. Barnes and Co., 1851.

Community Planning, Inc. and R. M. Towill Corp. *Master Plan for the Island of Maui.* Honolulu.

DAMON, ETHEL M. *Koamalu.* Vol. I. Honolulu, 1931. Privately printed.

DARLING, F. FRASER and JOHN P. MILTON (eds.). *Future Environments of North America.* Garden City, N.Y.: The Natural History Press, 1966.

DAY, ARTHUR GROVE. *Hawaii and its People.* New York: Meredith Press, 1968.

DEAN, ARTHUR L. *Alexander and Baldwin, Ltd. and the Predecessor Partnerships.* Honolulu: Alexander and Baldwin, Ltd., 1950.

DODGE, ERNEST S. *New England and the South Seas.* Cambridge: Harvard University Press, 1965.

DONDO, MATHURIN MARIUS. *Laperouse in Maui.* Wailuku, Hawaii: Maui Publishing Company, 1959.

"Evangelistic Tour of North Pacific Missionary Institute," *The Friend.* Honolulu: Hawaiian Board of Missions, January, 1901.

FINNEY, BEN R. and JAMES D. HOUSTON. *Surfing, the Sport of Hawaiian Kings.* Tokyo: Charles E. Tuttle Co., 1966.

FLEMING, MARTHA FOSS. *Old Trails of Maui.* Honolulu: William and Mary Alexander Chapter, Daughters of the American Revolution, 1933.

FORNANDER, ABRAHAM. *An Account of the Polynesian Race.* Vols. I, II, and III. London: Trübner and Co., 1878–1885.

FORSTER, JOHN. "Acculturation of Hawaiians on the Island of Maui, Hawaii." Unpublished thesis, University of California, Los Angeles, 1959.

———. "The Hawaiian Family System of Hana, Maui, 1957," *Journal of the Polynesian Society,* 162:2. Wellington, N.Z.: the Polynesian Society, Inc., June 1960.

FRASER, MABEL. "Agency-Plantation Histories." Unpublished notes and clippings. Hawaiian Sugar Planters' Association Library, Honolulu.

FUCHS, LAWRENCE H. *Hawaii Pono: A Social History.* New York: Harcourt, Brace and World, 1961.

GILMORE, A. B. *The Hawaiian Sugar Manual.* New Orleans: A. B. Gilmore, 1936–1951 passim.

"Haleakala Souvenir Edition," *Maui News,* February 23, 1935. Wailuku: Maui Publishing Co.

HAWAII AUDUBON SOCIETY. *Hawaii's Birds.* Honolulu: Hawaii Audubon Society, 1967.

Hawaiian Kingdom Statistical and Commercial Directory and Tourist's Guide. Honolulu, 1880–1881.

HEDEMANN, META M. "Hana from 1878." Unpublished manuscript.

"History of Sugar in Hana," *Pan-Pacific Journal.* Honolulu: Pan-Pacific Union, April-June 1940.

HOHMAN, ELMO PAUL. *The American Whaleman.* New York: Longmans, Green and Co., 1928.

HOWELL, MILTON and INEZ ASHDOWN. "Seven Sacred Pools of Kipahulu." Personal correspondence, Ulupalakua, Maui, 1968.

"Hundredth Anniversary Kaupo Huialoha Church, Anniversary Program," July 19, 1959. (In library of Dr. Milton Howell, Hana, Maui.)

ISE, JOHN. *Our National Park Policy: A Critical History.* Baltimore: Johns Hopkins Press (for Resources for the Future, Inc.), 1961.

"Jubilee Celebration of the Arrival of the Missionary Reinforcement of 1837." Honolulu: Hawaiian Mission Children's Society, 1887.

"Kaeleku Sugar Company," *Evening Bulletin.* Honolulu, 1909.

"Kaeleku Sugar Company," *Honolulu Star-Bulletin,* Panama Canal Number (Industrial Section), Honolulu, April 1882.

KAMAKAU, SAMUEL M. *Ruling Chiefs of Hawaii.* Honolulu: The Kamehameha Schools Press, 1961.

KITSON, ARTHUR. *Captain James Cook, "The Circumnavigator."* New York: E. P. Dutton, 1907.

KUYKENDALL, RALPH S. *The Hawaiian Kingdom,* Vols, I, II, and III. Honolulu: University of Hawaii Press, 1968.

"Labor Committee Report," *The Planters Monthly,* April 1882. Published by the Planters' Labor and Supply Co., Honolulu.

"Letters from Mr. Conde dated Hana 12/15/41 and 11/1/45," *The Missionary Herald.* Boston: American Board of Commissioners for Foreign Missions, 1841 (Vol. XXXVII) and 1846 (Vol. XLII).

LIND, ANDREW W. *Hawaii's People.* Honolulu: University of Hawaii Press, 1967.

LUOMALA, KATHARINE. "Maui-of-a-Thousand-Tricks," *Bernice P. Bishop Museum Bulletin* 198. Honolulu: Bishop Museum, 1949.

———. *Voices on the Wind.* Honolulu: Bishop Museum Press, 1955.

McDONALD, SHOEMAKER. "Strategic" War-Winning Rubber of Hawaii. Honolulu: Paradise of the Pacific, July 1939 and August 1939.

MALO, DAVID. *Hawaiian Antiquities.* Honolulu: Hawaiian Gazette Co., 1903.

MAUDE, H. E. "The Gilbert and Ellice Islands," *Pan-Pacific Journal,* Honolulu: Pan-Pacific Union, July-September, 1941.

"Maui Plantations," Centenary Number, *Honolulu Star-Bulletin,* April 1920.

MEDEIROS, JOSEPHINE K. "Story of the Seven Sacred Pools of Kipahulu Valley." Unpublished manuscript (mimeo.), Hotel Hana-Maui, Hana, 1960.

MELLEN, KATHLEEN DICKENSON. *The Lonely Warrior—The Life and Times of Kamehameha the Great of Hawaii.* New York: Hastings House, 1949.

NEWTON, I. C. (ed.). *Who's Who of the Counties of Maui and Kauai.* Wailuku, Hawaii: L. C. Newton and John A. Lee.

OLMSTED, MRS. NILS KALELEOKALANI. "Na Wahi Pana O Hana." Unpublished manuscript. In Maui Public Library.

PLEASANT, E. E. "The Hana Mission Station." Unpublished manuscript. In Maui Public Library.

"Report of Captain Tierney," *The Planters Monthly,* February 1883. Honolulu: Planters' Labor and Supply Company.

"Report of the Missionaries at Lahaina, 10-15-1828," *Missionary Herald,* XXV:212, July 1829.

RUHEN, OLAF. *Harpoon in my Hand.* Australia: Angus and Robertson, 1966.

SCHMITT, ROBERT C. and ROSE C. STROMBEL. "Marriage and Divorce in Hawaii before 1870," *Hawaii Historical Review,* II:2, January 1966 (mimeo.)

SIMONDS, WILLIAM A. *The Hawaiian Telephone Story*. Honolulu: Hawaiian Telephone Co., 1958.

STEARNS, HAROLD T. *Geology of the State of Hawaii*. Palo Alto: Pacific Books, 1966.

THRUM, THOMAS G. (ed.). *Hawaiian Almanac and Annual*. Honolulu: Thrum and Oat, 1875-1932 *passim*.

U.S. DEPARTMENT OF THE INTERIOR, National Park Service. *Administration Policies for Natural Areas of the National Park System*. Washington, D.C., 1967.

Voyage Round the World Performed in the Years 1785, 1787, and 1788, by the Boussole and Astrolabe, under the Command of J. F. G. De Laperhouse. London: Lackington, Allen and Co., 1807.

WARNER, RICHARD E. (ed.). *Scientific Report of the Kipahulu Valley Expedition*. San Francisco: The Nature Conservancy, 1968.

WATSON, LESLIE J. "Old Hawaiian Land Huis—Their Development and Dissolution." Unpublished manuscript. Honolulu, December 1932. In University of Hawaii Library.

WENKAM, ROBERT. "Annie Pak Chong and Frank Decoite." Tape-recorded interview, Hamoa, Maui, Hawaii, March 19, 1968.

———. "Annie Smith and Elizabeth Haia." Tape-recorded interview, Kipahulu, Maui, Hawaii, March 17, 1968.

———. "Nick Soon." Tape-recorded interview, Kaupo, Maui, Hawaii, March 17, 1968.

WILFONG, GEORGE. "Twenty Years' Experience in Cane Culture," *The Planters Monthly*, October 1882. Honolulu: Planters' Labor and Supply Co.

YZENDOORN, REGINALD. *History of the Catholic Mission in the Hawaiian Islands*, Honolulu: Honolulu Star-Bulletin, 1927.

GLOSSARY OF HAWAIIAN PLANTS AND TREES

Ahinahina (Silversword), *Arhyroxiphium sandwicense*. Native Hawaiian plant growing only in Haleakala and high mountain slopes of Hawaii island. The silversword blooms once then dies.

Ama'u-ma'u (fern), *Sadleria cyatheoides*. Brownish soft growth at base of fronds used to stuff pillows and mattresses. Pith of trunk eaten during famines and used as trim on lauhala houses.

Ape'ape, *Gunnera petaloidea*.

'Awa, *Piper methysticum*. Ground-up root juices used as ceremonial drink throughout the Pacific.

'Awaapuhi Ke'oke'o (white ginger), *Hedychium coronarium*.

'Awaapuhi Melemele (yellow ginger), *Hedychium flavum*.

Foa (ironwood), *Casuarina equisetifolia*.

Hala (screw pine), *Pandanus odoratissimus*. Native of Hawaii and other Pacific islands. Leaves are dried and cut into narrow strips for weaving "lauhala" floor mats, bags, and sandals for walking on rough lava trails.

Haole koa, *Leucaena glauca*. Used for cattle fodder and seed leis.

Haole pamakani, *Eupatorium glandulosum*.

Hapu (tree fern), *Cibotium chamissoi*. The silky base of the fronds is the "pulu" exported by early Hawaiians for stuffing mattresses.

Hau, *Hibiscus tiliaceus*. The thin bark is dried and stripped to make "grass" hula skirts. Grown over supports, the twisting branches interlock and form arbor shelters. Used for canoe outriggers.

'Iliahi (Haleakala sandalwood), *Santalum haleakalae*. Used for aromatic chests and temple incense in the Orient.

——— Jacaranda, *Jacaranda acutifolia*.

Kalo (taro), *Colocasia esculenta*. Staple food of the Hawaiians made into a paste (poi). Brought to Hawaii by Polynesians on their earliest voyages. Dry and wetland varieties; some forms favored for tasty leaves. Wetland taro grown in flooded terraces (lo'i). Black mud of taro patches used to dye tapa patterns.

Kamani (tropical almond), *Terminalia catappa*. The reddish wood was used for houses and the bark, leaves, and roots were for tanning skins and native remedies.

Kauila, *Alphitonia ponderosa*. Rare native tree of extremely hard, heavy wood that sinks in water. Used for spears and tapa design beaters.

Kawa'u (Hawaiian holly), *Ilex anomala*.

Kiawe (mesquite), *Prosopis chilensis*. Extensively used for charcoal; the seed pods are excellent cattle food.

Ko (sugar cane), *Saccharum officinarum*. Introduced by first Polynesians. Planted for sugar and house thatch.

Koa, *Acacia koa*. Used for canoes, calabashes, and surfboards, and in recent years for ukuleles and finished cabinet work.

Kolea, *Suttonia lessertiana*. Hawaiians used the charcoal for tapa dye and the logs for beating tapa.

Kuawa (guava), *Psidium guajava*.

Kukui (candlenut tree), *Aleurites moluccana*. Native tree common throughout Hawaii. Raw nuts are an excellent cathartic; oil is burned in stone lamps; roots yield black tapa dye; polished nuts are made into decorative leis.

Ie'ie, *Freycinetia arborea*. Native vine considered sacred, used along with other woods to build the hula altar for Laka, goddess of the hula. The long aerial roots were sometimes split and used for weaving baskets, calabash slings, and helmets.

Mai'a (banana), *Musa (spp.)*. Many varieties introduced by early Polynesians.

Manako (mango), *Mangifera indica*.

Mau'u (sedge).

Ni'ani'au (swordfern), *Nephrolepis exaltata*.

Niu (coconut palm), *Cocos nucifera*. Nut used for food, drinking, soap, and twine; palm leaves woven into thatch.

'Ohe (bamboo), *Schizostachyum (spp.)*. Believed introduced from Tahiti. Grows in dense forests, excluding other plants, reaching over 15 feet. Many uses, including fish poles, knives, nose flutes, dance percussion wands, canoe outriggers, building posts; split for mats; young shoots cooked and eaten.

Olona, *Touchardia latifolia*. Bark woven into fish nets and sail rigging.

Ohia Lehua, *Metrosideros collina*. Hawaiians used the very hard wood for idols and spears. Common Hawaiian forest tree, famous in legend and chant. "Lehua" was the name given to the first man killed in battle.

Panini (cactus), *Opuntia megacantha*. Introduced from Mexico about 1800. Hawaiians fermented a drink from the edible fruit. The name means "very unfriendly."

Pili, *Heteropogon contortus*. Commonly used for grass-house walls and roof. In dry areas a pili house may last ten years.

Piliuka (bunchgrass), *Deschampsia australis forma haleakalenis*.

Ti, *Cordyline terminalis*. Important plant to the early Hawaiians; leaves used for house thatch, raincoats, food wrappers, and Hukilau fishing nets. A brandy called okolehao is made from the fermented root. In battle, a stalk of ti was displayed to signal surrender.

Ulu (breadfruit), *Artocarpus incisus*. Carried by the first Polynesians from Tahiti. Bark used for tapa. Sap used to patch canoe hulls. Staple food.

Uluhe (false staghorn), *Dicranopteris linearis*.

Wilelaiki (Christmas berry), *Schinus terebinthifolius*.

Wiliwili, *Erythrina monosperma*.

Wiliwili (false wiliwili; red sandalwood), *Adenanthera pavonina*. Native tree. The bright red seeds are used in leis.

that continuing income from the property can be assured only if scenic assets and cultural traditions are preserved. If Hana Ranch succeeds in its plan, it will become a model for all Hawaii.

Ranch consultant Edward Brownlee writes that, "The Hana coast, with its large proportion of Hawaiian people, remains a last chance, with the tools of sound economic and physical planning, to encourage the preservation and viable continuance of the Hawaiian culture." Hana planners will be working within self-imposed limitations in laying out a golf course, designing a new Hasegawa General Store, and building residential condominiums in which mainlanders and Hawaiian workers will live together. The ranch gates from Hana to Kipahulu are now, and will remain, unlocked. "Kapu" signs are gone and the pastures are open for picnics, swimming, or a night of fishing. A great part of the Hana pastureland will never be developed, and all of the forest land will remain forever wild.

POPULATION. A system of parks, zoning ordinances, easements, and a sensible parkway will be little more than holding actions if Hawaii's tourist population continues to grow unchecked. The area of Haleakala National Park may be doubled and the number of county beach parks tripled, but corresponding increases in tourist populations will ruin Maui. The impact of cheap tour groups flown to Hawaii by superjet, housed in low-cost hotels and bussed about to hasty views less satisfying than a postcard, should not be Maui's fate. There is no democracy in crushing an island's beauty for all the future under the weight of a mass of tourists who only glimpse the beauty as it passes.

The master plan for Maui must find a means for keeping resident and tourist populations within the carrying capacity of the landscape. There is an optimum population for Maui, and we must soon decide what it is. The decision must be made before it is too late—before scenic drives are lost to freeways, before the old churches at Kipahulu, Keanae, and Kaupo are lost in the hearts of tourist ghettos. Soon County planners will have to decide how many people will be allowed to visit Maui, stay overnight, walk the trails, and drive the highways. Soon the County will have to decide when hotel-building permits will no longer be issued, and state land-use commissioners will have to call an end to urban expansion by freezing urban boundary lines. If these decisions are made now, and not made piecemeal, but as part of a larger plan, Maui will be a better place for it.

The growth of tourism anticipated in the next years will require wise implementation of Hawaii's land-use laws. New resorts and hotels must be firmly directed to areas where the least damage to scenic resources will occur. Absentee hotel developers and private landowners will not direct this growth in the best interests of Hawaii's future. Only citizen commissioners who understand that corporate profit is only a part of the people's interest, and for whom the enlightened land laws of Hawaii are clearly in mind, can be trusted with Maui's future.

Hawaii leads the nation in master planning for land. In 1964 the State zoned all its lands, placing them in urban, rural, agricultural, or conservation districts—a tremendously difficult, but enlightened undertaking. Now planners from California and other states with growth problems are turning to the Pacific to discover how Hawaii does it. Hawaii should retain this leadership in land management. If, as David Brower writes, "we need new patterns: not for growth, not for blind progress, but for equilibrium between man and his finite environment, an environment that must stay alive if man is to stay alive"—then those patterns should continue to come from Hawaii. "The regulation of technology," writes Wilbur H. Ferry, Vice President of Fund for the Republic, "is the most important intellectual and political task on the American agenda." That regulation of technology can begin in Hawaii. The State has done well, but should not be complacent. It is time for another farsighted environmental protection plan, on East Maui this time. Hawaii should again be a model for the nation.

The land of East Maui has been treated roughly. The native Hawaiians did not do badly by the land in their first centuries on it, but when asked to, they bargained it away for credit at the company store. The missionaries, who never liked it for what it was, spent long years imagining how much like New England it might someday be. The sugar planters simplified its plant and animal complexity and made fortunes from it; the cattlemen fed it to their steers and shipped them to market. Now we can do better by it.

Maui has a slogan, *Maui No Ka Oe*—Maui the best of all. We must utilize every talent and innovative skill to keep Maui the best. We must not confuse growth with progress. We must use more efficiently the space we already occupy, and plan more wisely for the space we have not yet altered. Our success will not lie in how much money we make from the land, or even in the number of visitors we contrive to have enjoy its beauty, but in how well we preserve it. The visitor fifty years from now will best judge our custodianship of the Maui land we hold in trust.

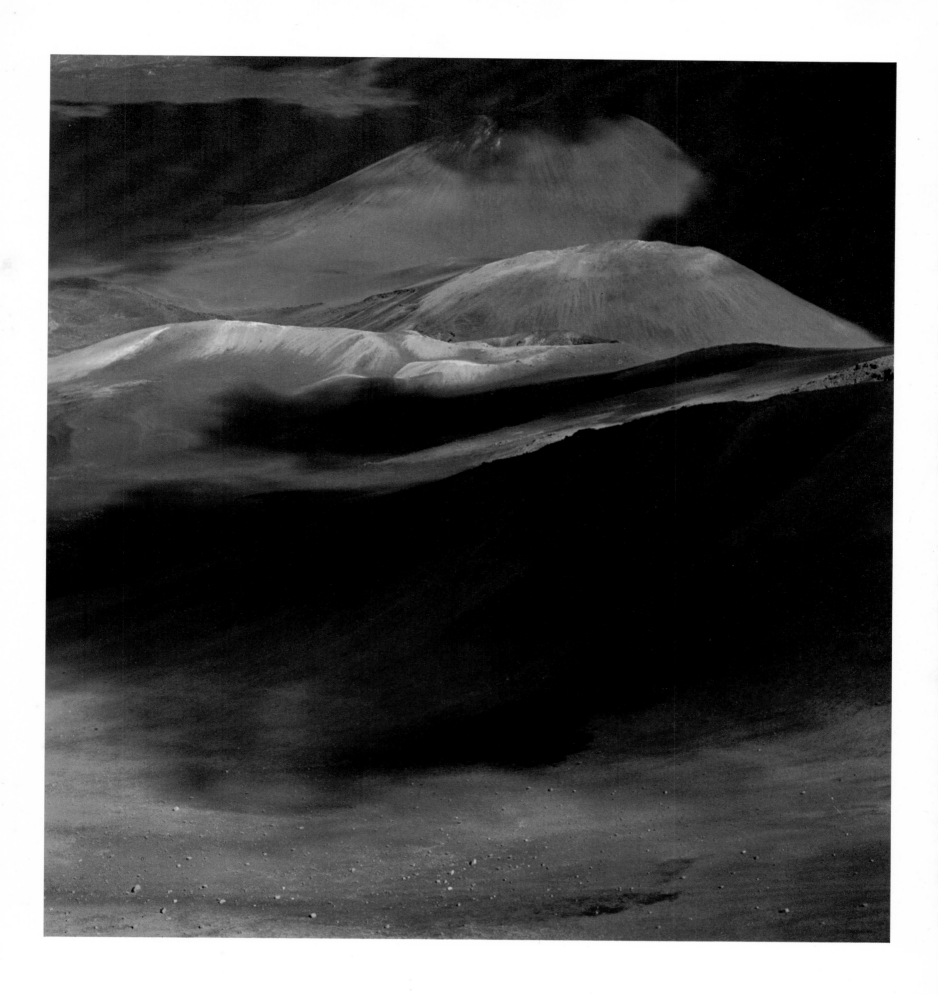

RAIN SONGS

Let the rain fall, for rain is good.
It patters down, it pelts down,
It flattens the forest growth,
It sprinkles musically on the lehua.
The lehua trees blossom, the yellow lehua,
When the rain comes to the lehua of Kailua.
The lehua petals are heavy with raindrops,
Heavy, heavy and full-blown.

Waterfall, Hana Road

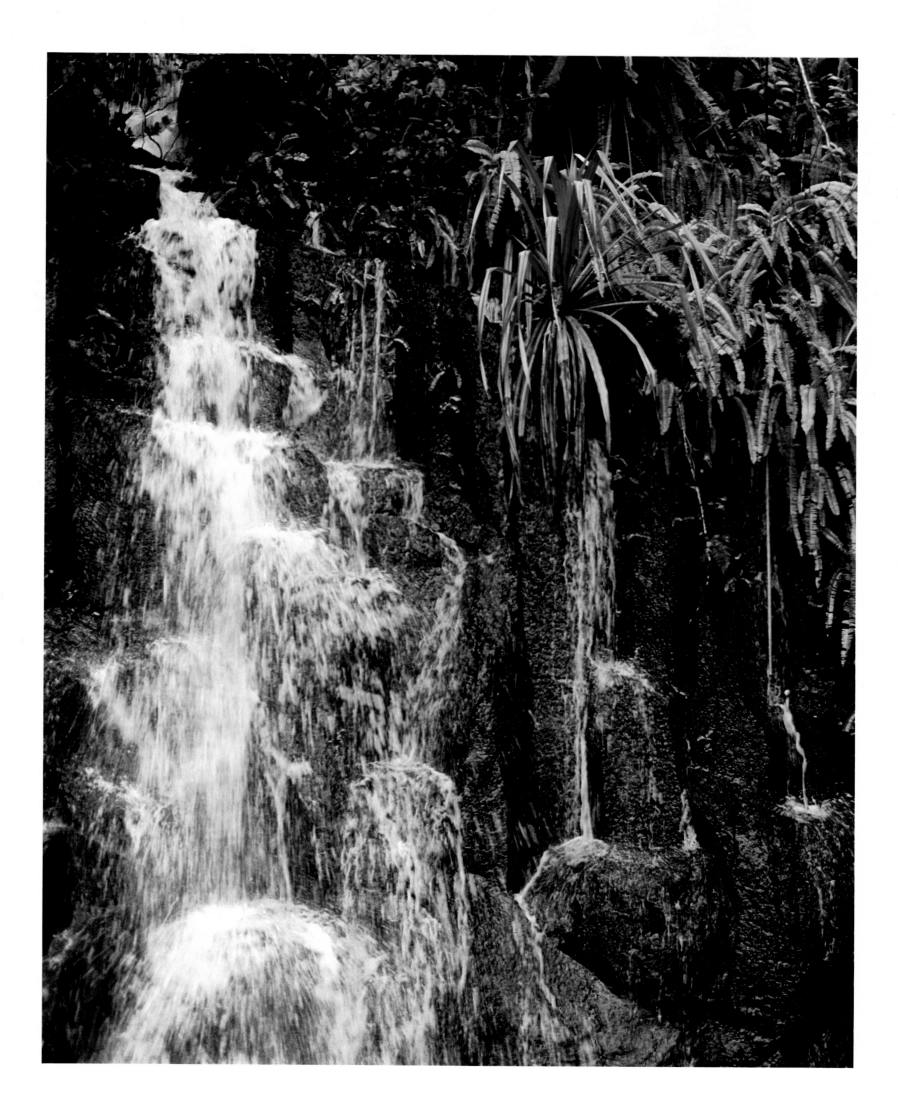

The rain that brings out the full-blown flowers,
And draws them close down to the shore.
The rain goes out to sea,
It falls on Hawini like teardrops,
It passes along over the capes,
It creeps by the cliffs and capes,
Creeps by the cape of Mokupapa.
The rain comes uninvited.

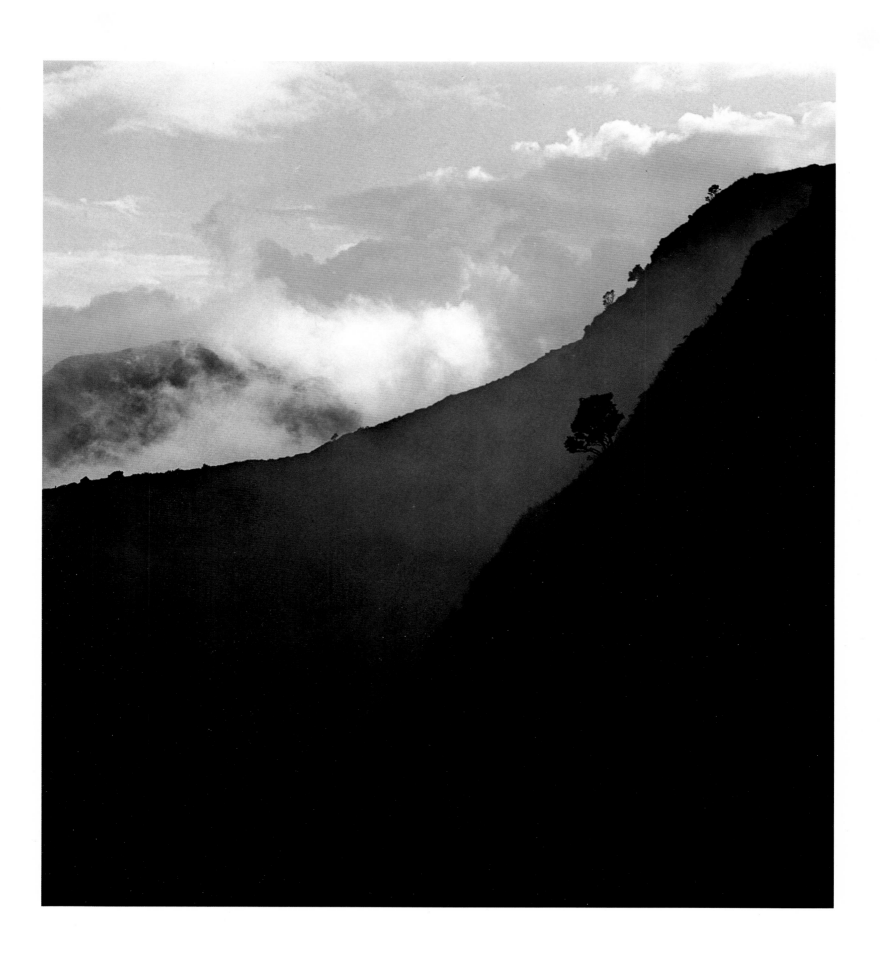

The rain patters on the roofs of the sleeping houses,
Then it dances away to the forest.
Quietly fell the rain in the forest,
Whirling came the rain in the forest,
The rain in the forest twisted this way and that,
Drop by drop fell the rain in the forest,
Mist-like fell the rain in the forest,
Chilly was the rain in the forest,
The rain in the forest was cold,
The rain in the forest chilled through to the bone,
The rain in the forest made one shiver,
The rain in the forest ripened the mountain apples.

Ohia lehua forest, Kipahulu Valley

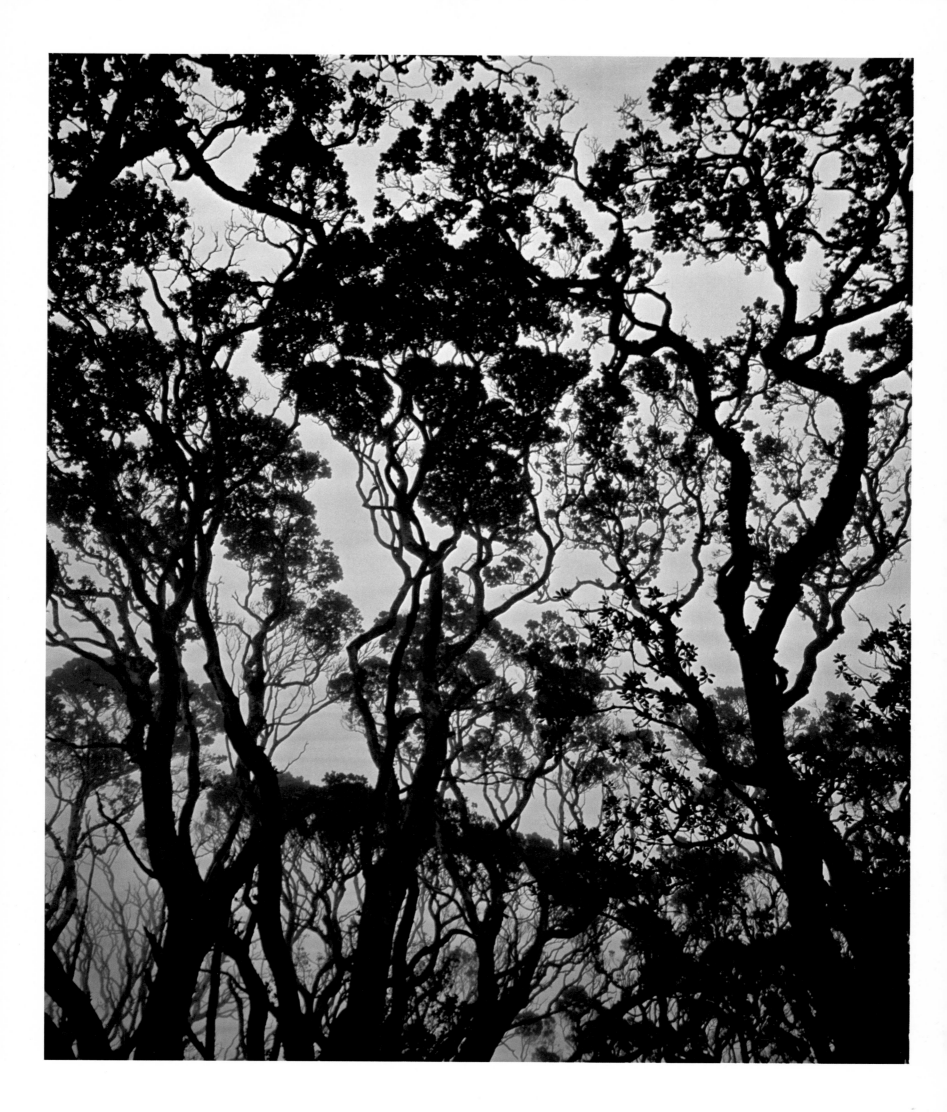

They two wandered in the forest,
To the rootless koa tree at Kahini-kolo.
Fern leaves were woven into loin cloths,
Ti leaves were broken off and worn on the back,
Thus were we clothed,
Wandering, wandering on,
Wandering and living on the ripe fruit of the pandanus.
Thus passed our days of hunger, O my companion,
Through the pouring rain, the wind-blown rain,
The ceaselessly pouring rain,
Through much heavy rain, through light rain, until the rain ceased.

There we were till the rain ceased falling, O my companion,
My companion in the hurrying whirlwind . . .
Rain that came from the lowlands,
Rain that came from the east,
Rain that came from the south,
Rain that came from above,
Rain that came from below,
Along the cape of Pu'upaoa, overgrown with pandanus,
There was the rain that pelted the pandanus fruit,
Drenching the sand where the sand eels fed,
The eels that ate the pandanus of Mahamoku,
The rain that ripened the mountain apples of Wai'oli.
I was glad that you were my lord.

—recorded and translated from the Hawaiian by
SAMUEL KAMAKAU

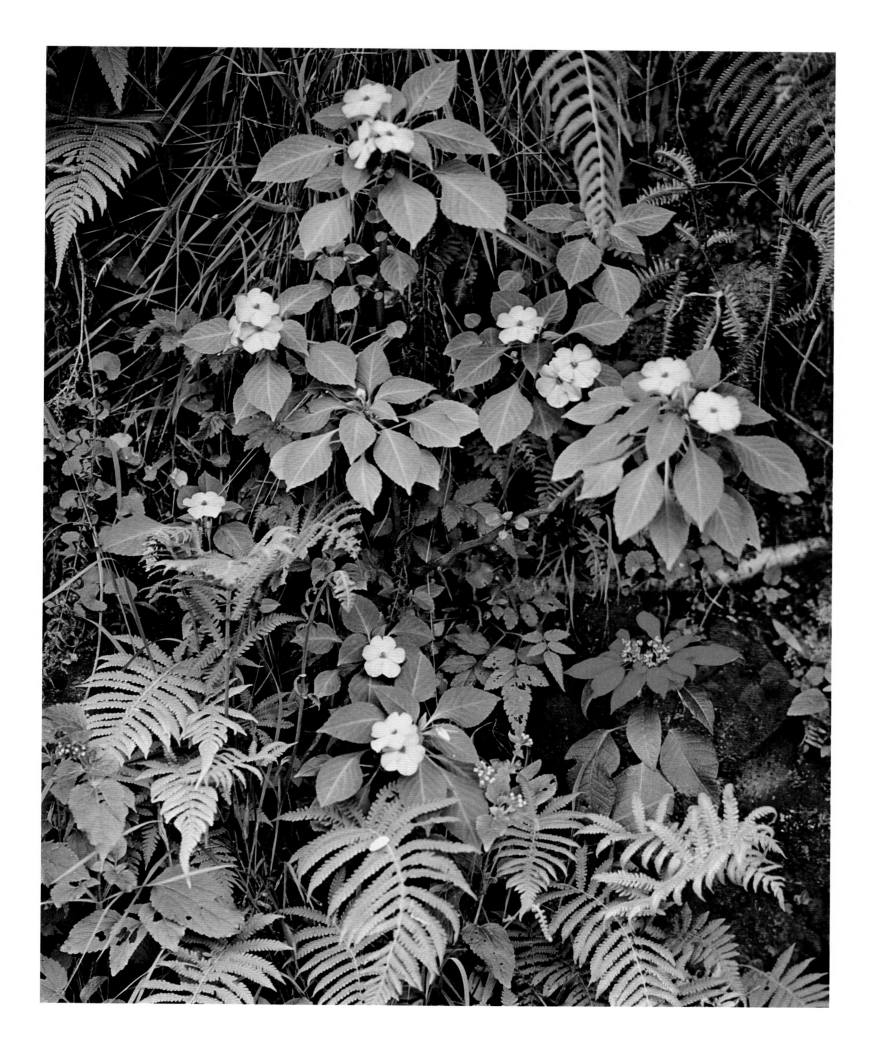

KIPAHULU SKETCHES

by Kenneth Brower

Kipahulu is a fan of old lava that begins thinly at the mouth of a valley high on Maui's side and spreads in a steep descent to the sea. The eruption that pushed out the fan was an ancient one, and the slopes of Kipahulu are now green. The fan today is cattle country. Much of it has been cleared for pasture—rather, is continually being cleared, for the soil is so rich, the rainfall so heavy, that it takes the concerted effort of cattle and ranch hands to keep the thickets from returning.

A Hawaiian civilization and later a sugar-producing civilization of Oriental laborers and white overseers were once established here, but have left few traces. Today the Hawaiians are back, but in small numbers. You can walk the length of the Kipahulu road without seeing anyone. The country lies open to the high cumulus clouds that pass on bright days over the island. On darker days it's a country of sudden squalls and rainbows, a good country for walking in rain and sunshine at the same time, or for pausing under a tree as a squall passes over, then walking out to watch the squall continue down the coast, darkening farther pastures. It's a country of lean dogs without collars. It's a country of plover who stand sentinels in the grass until you draw near, then flee to skim the undulating pasture as they would skim the surface of the sea.

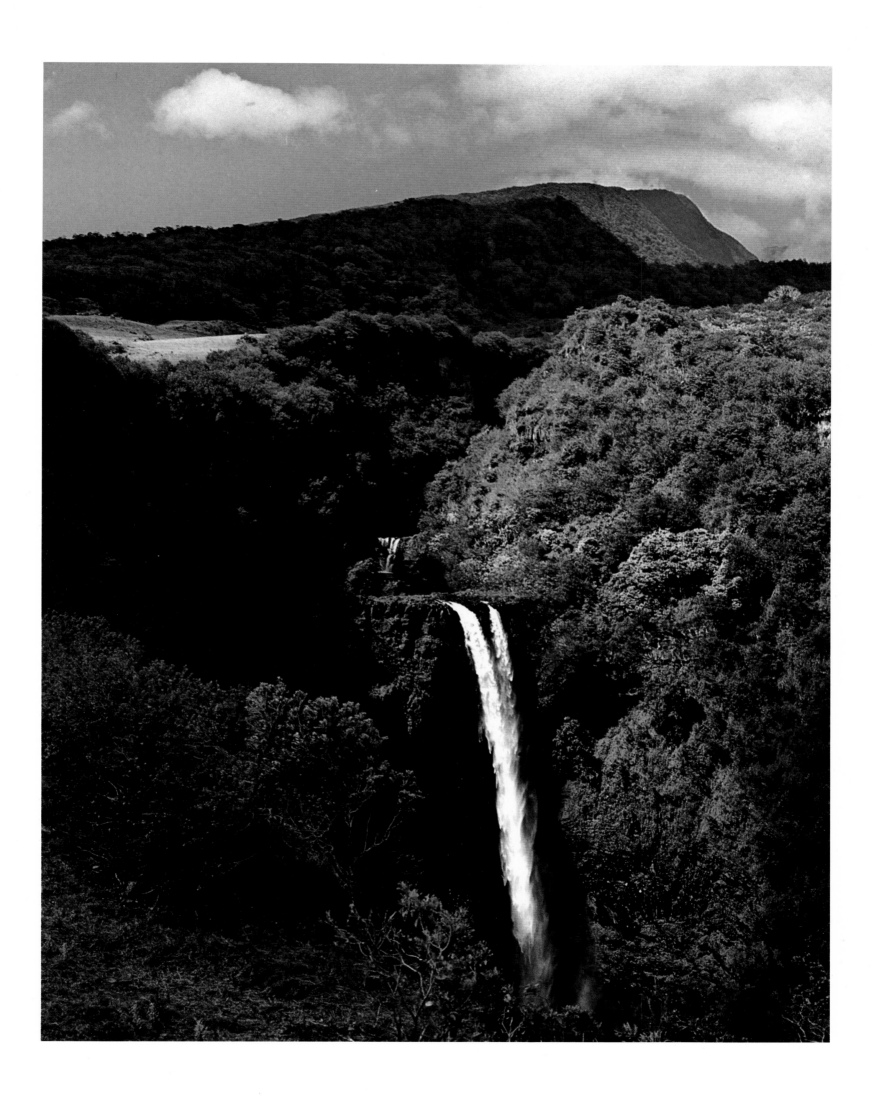

The following are sketches of the people of Kipahulu. The sketches are brief, for the people don't talk much about themselves or their neighbors, and don't reveal much. The idea of interchange of personality is a novel idea for Kipahulu residents, and not very interesting to them. But the sketches are important to a book on Maui's parkland because the people are part of the land. When the boundaries of Haleakala National Park were extended to include Kipahulu the people there became features of the Park.

Only Kipahulu biographies are included here, though there are many other people on East Maui of park caliber. No mention is made of Leilani, a large brown lady with a full neck and bright red lipstick who lives farther up the coast. No mention is made of Leilani's house, scant and neat and painted green, lost in the breadfruit and banana trees, in the passionfruit vines, in the wide lawns and gardens that surround it. It was hot the day we visited her, and Leilani's son brought us beer from the house. He brought bottles for the men and a glass for the lady lawyer who was with us. The glass was overfull, and the son did not hold it carefully. Beer spilled off his hand as he walked toward us. Leilani spoke sharply to him, and he righted the glass.

Leilani's old mother showed us through the garden, and we followed with our beer. The fertility of the soil was such that the flowers of the garden were deliberately grown on rocky patches in the lawn. The soil itself offered too fertile a hold for weeds. Leilani's mother gave the lady lawyer a human chest plant, potted in a rusty tin can. It was called a chest plant, the grandmother said, because the ribbing of the leaf made it look like the X-ray of a human chest. She gave the rest of us some airplant, called so, she said, because it lives on nothing but air. In her garden it grew hanging from a very inorganic and clearly non-nutritive piece of insulated wire. When I politely doubted the airplant, the grandmother tugged off some more of it and pushed the evidence at me. But none of this is mentioned; nothing of the dogs, the lawn, the old cars parked about, the bright masses of flowers, the cold beer, the grandmother and her pure Polynesian features, the shirtless, brown, friendly sons, the palms, the surf sounding below, or the blue ocean spread out before us.

And not everyone in Kipahulu is included here. Joe, who drives the Kipahulu Ranch tractor, is not. He had hundreds of fairy tales to tell, he said, but he always found a reason for not telling them. Nor is the history of Kipahulu's old Eskimo woman included. This boreal lady's haole husband nailed her in a crate, they say, and slipped below deck every night to feed her on her long passage from Alaska. She arrived in the Hawaiian Islands a stowaway. Her husband has since died, her children have grown up and departed. She is now a quiet woman, and spends much of her time alone. I remember her sitting above the Seven Pools, under a pandanus tree, in a litter of pandanus nuts, watching a Hawaiian family swim below. Little could her mother have guessed the lands she would travel in.

Age has a way of reconciling racial differences, and the Eskimo lady at first glance looks Hawaiian, but she has never learned to be fluent in any of the tongues of her adopted country. She must have a story to tell, if one knew the language to ask her in.

The people of the sketches that follow live on an isolated part of the East Maui coast. They wake and sleep in pastoral country at the foot of Kipahulu's great and only partly explored valley. Though they are only a half hour from the small town of Hana, and though they drive there often to shop, to go to school, to the movie, or to work, still at night they go home. As the road home from Hana enters Kipahulu, the pavement worsens and the residents have to slow down. If they stop and turn off their lights, the Hawaiian night is lightless again, except for the stars. The people of Kipahulu sleep, then, and wake, on the edge of civilization, and are less involved with it than their nearest neighbors are.

There are no Yick Lung vending machines in Kipahulu, or anything like them.

Yick Lung Co.
Candies seeds   *Superior quality*
Sweet sour seeds
Shredded Mango
Li Hing Mui
Lemon bits
Whole seed
Sweet wet seed
Pistachio Nuts
Whole Apricots

All fruit in Kipahulu comes from trees. In Hana there is an art class, but Kipahulu does not have one.

The art class is taught by John Picard, a Southerner who has only recently come to Maui. Picard specializes in painting beaches. He sells enough of his paintings, and enrolls enough art students—for the most part retired mainlanders and older Hawaiian working people—to get by. Picard loves Maui and is delighted that he is able to make his living there by painting. He holds his class at night in one of Hana School's classrooms. He leaves the door open, for the Hana nights are warm.

While Picard's students work, the Hana boys and girls who have lingered after school laugh and talk on the long porch outside the door. There is no other place for high-school people to hang out after dark, and they stay at the school for hours. The conversations on the porch are subdued. The young people are easier in the company of the other sex than people their age on the mainland. The jokes from the porch are unstrained, the laughter easy.

Occasionally someone from the porch will come inside and look over an artist's shoulder. Sometimes a wrestler will take a break from wrestling practice in the next bungalow and will enter in his sweat clothes to check on an artist's progress. But no one stays long. The observers expect no surprises from the art class, apparently, and in evenings past have formed lasting opinions of the various talents in it. They look perfunctorily and wander off.

Picard moves lightly among his students. He has short graying hair and a short goatee. He is a slender man in faded blue jeans and white shirt, and moves gracefully. He leans over a great Hawaiian woman and gives her instructions. She sits at her desk smiling and listening—great back and neck, unblemished expanse of smooth brown shoulder above her bright red, flowery muumuu, hair black and beautiful, with a white flower in it, head lowered and attentive. Picard is thin and colorless, but still graceful, beside her.

Picard addresses the class with a deep Southern accent. "You ought to get you some paper talls," he tells one student. "You have raw umbah?" he asks another. "Raw umbah looks good on rocks." Picard's dialect has a few locutions in common with Hawaii's pidgin, but not enough, and communication is a problem. It may be one reason that the class pays little attention to its teacher.

I had not been watching the class long my first night there, when a bald, heavy man walked over and introduced himself. He had been in the garment industry in Pasadena, he told me, and had later owned a private hospital, but was now retired. "I daub in painting and photography," he said. He conceded that he wasn't any good at it, but left some room for doubt.

As we watched Picard, the man who had been in the garment industry told me about his life in Hana. He told me about his boat, about the size of his orchid house, about what he had done for the community. He was talkative, good natured, and delighted with things. When he had first come to Hana, he said, he tried to organize a youth program. He had noticed that the kids had nothing to do after school, and that the girls got pregnant. If they had something to do, he reasoned, it would be different. It was just energy, after all, wasn't it?

The man from the garment industry usually participated in the class, but tonight he was just observing. It was clearly the role he preferred. He enjoyed watching the people. He indicated each of the students with a nod, and told me who they were. This woman was secretary to the manager of Hana Ranch. That man was a postman. This woman was a housekeeper. That man worked at Hasegawa General Store.

Directly in front of us was a powerful Hawaiian in shorts, a worker at the hotel, my informant whispered. The man had calves that looked to be carved from blocks of some dark Hawaiian hardwood. He seemed cramped by the desk, but he worked with intense concentration. His wife, sitting on the next desk, watched with admiration.

Everyone in the class was painting the same scene, working from a Picard beach painting at the front of the class. They looked up from time to time to check their accuracy. Picard continued to move from student to student. He would sometimes stop and sit down, take the drawing board in hand, and point out errors. He did not mind picking up a palette knife and making the corrections himself. One man, a heavy-set, retired mainlander, objected to Picard's method. "I'm not trying to imitate you, now," the man said. He was defending his rights—speaking up for his own vision—but he didn't sound very sure of himself, and Picard moved on to the next student. "That's not earth green," Picard said. "I said to use *earth* green here. This is much too green." He moved on again, leaning over the next student's shoulder. "Here, mix you some of this," he said.

But Kipahulu people are not part of this. A Kipahulu boy might be among the wrestlers who drop in on the class, but he is soon on his way home, his car filled with friends, tired friends whom he drops off one at a time until only Kipahulu boys are left, one or two of them, and the final miles pass without much talking, these last boys knowing each other so well, the car's headlights illuminating giant toads on the road, illuminating briefly the grotto with the white stone Virgin and latest offering of flowers, illuminating the green sign that commemorates an event in the life of Helio Koaeloa, who long ago converted this coast to Catholicism, illuminating finally the home gate.

A Kipahulu mother might attend the class if flowers, shells, bottles, and driftwood were not so readily at hand and so much more satisfactory than canvas and oil. The society of the art class—of the retired capitalists, ranch secretaries, and store clerks—has as little appeal for her as for her son.

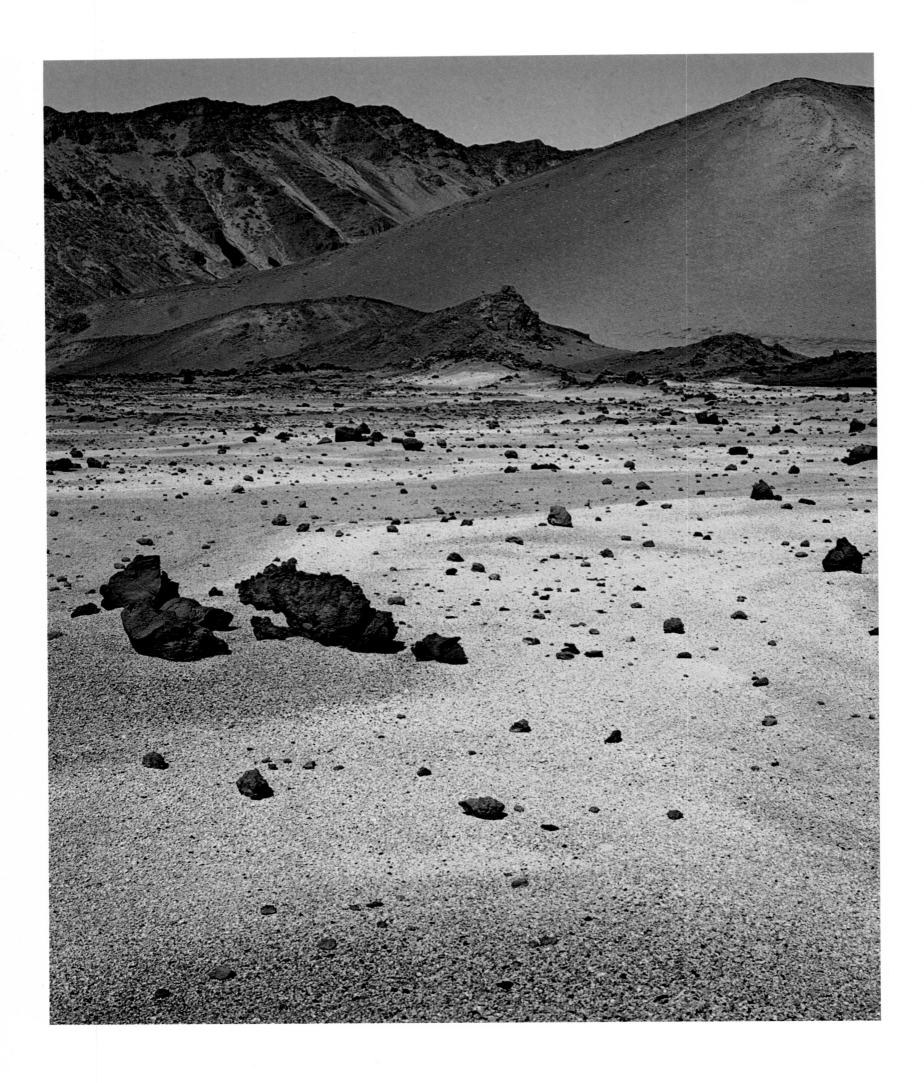

Kipahulu people are in the habit of moving a quarter of a mile from their homes to live their weekends in tents by the sea. To an outsider it might seem more sensible to walk the quarter mile each morning and return at night to the comfort of home, but it does not seem so to the Hawaiians of Kipahulu. They inhabit a confined land, and enjoy living freely on it. They move about with the boundaried rootlessness of a migratory people who have reached their last island.

Kipahulu sons, unlike the young men of the Azores, the Galápagos, the Aran Islands, or other of the planet's more barren archipelagos, have no burning desire to leave and see the world. Some do leave, but many stay. Their apparent lack of curiosity might seem lamentable in young descendants of such renowned wanderers. But Kipahulu boys have all seen Honolulu at least once, and they understand the nature of cities. They have seen movies, and now television, and know what the rest of the world promises. They have weighed their island against this, and have decided not to risk what they have. It is strange to hear them, the newest generation of a race of gamblers, extoll Kipahulu's quiet when they have known little else. They speak from an informed innocence possible only in our age perhaps, but it still sometimes seems that the Mediterranean men who described Adam did not make a true character—that the mistake for which we remember the first resident of Paradise was an unlikely mistake.

The country that holds imaginations so recently nomadic is pastureland, but the pasture is never tiresome. It has its hidden places. On the stream that feeds Seven Pools there is a tiny dam, and behind the dam, a pool. The pool takes several turns as the stream canyon turns, then ends a hundred yards above the dam, where the stream flows freely again. The canyon is narrow and its walls are high and steep. There is a partial canopy of trees above, and little light gets through. The surface of the pool is dark, and light falls only in patches. Mosquitos breed in small pools below the dam, in such numbers that while he undresses a swimmer must walk briskly back and forth on the narrow dam. Once in the water, however, he is free of the mosquitos. The water is cool and clear. Everywhere on the bottom of the pool are guavas, fallen from the trees above. They are ghostly golden in deep water and bright yellow in shallow water where the patches of sunlight fall. As you enter, you expect the water to taste a bit of decay, for the pool is still and the fallen guavas everywhere, but the water is fresh as spring water.

The country that holds the descendants of the Marquesans and of the Sandwich Islanders who shipped out in the whaleships of Melville's time is a country of great mango trees. They stand here and there in Kipahulu's pastures, their leaves growing densely, the ground beneath them shady and bare, the bare places smelling of the cattle who rest there in the middle of the day.

It's a country of mongooses, lately of Asia but adaptable and part of the country now. They are animated tails, quickly disappearing tails, tails with pointed noses that start from the grass at the edge of the pavement and bound close to the ground, rapidly across the road.

It's a country without real seasons or much range of temperature, a country that might be monotonous if it were not for the changes that water brings. Rainstorms are always moving west across the ocean, darkening here and there the sometimes blue, sometimes metal-colored plane. Inland, the high ridges are always interesting for the mist plays a thousand different games. One valley will hold a rainstorm and be ghostly, the next will lie inviting in the sun. It's a country of double rainbows and of squalls that come quick over the hill, the fine drops surprising you in the sunshine. It's a country of clear, quiet streams that change, after a night of rain, to tea-colored rivers that are unrecognizable.

It's a country that might even then be monotonous if it were not for the great, almost impenetrable, and largely unexplored valley above. Every Kipahulu boy has hunted pigs in the lower reaches of Kipahulu Valley, and many Kipahulu girls have foraged there. Many of the boys, as porters, have been a considerable distance up the valley's west ridge. They have felt the temperature drop as they climbed, until at Camp II the cold thin air seemed unnatural for Hawaii. They have climbed into the lower branches of the koa that overlooks the valley at Camp I. Below on the valley floor is a sea of koa, so far below that the lacework of white branches against the green is only just perceptible.

The canopy of trees protects you from the wind that blows out of the valley, but once in the branches of the solitary koa you are exposed to it. The wind rises in the middle of a hush, and smoothly, with perfect graduation, gains speed. There is no gustiness, just a featureless wall of wind that grows weightier, a smooth and general acceleration. When the wind blows its hardest, there is nothing mild or Hawaiian about it. It is something to remember afterward, when you are down on Kipahulu's coast. It must make things easier when Kipahulu's pastures seem tame.

The following are sketches of a life that is something like the old Hawaiian life. If we plan well, protecting Maui from overpopulation and overuse, there will always be stories like these to tell. —KENNETH BROWER

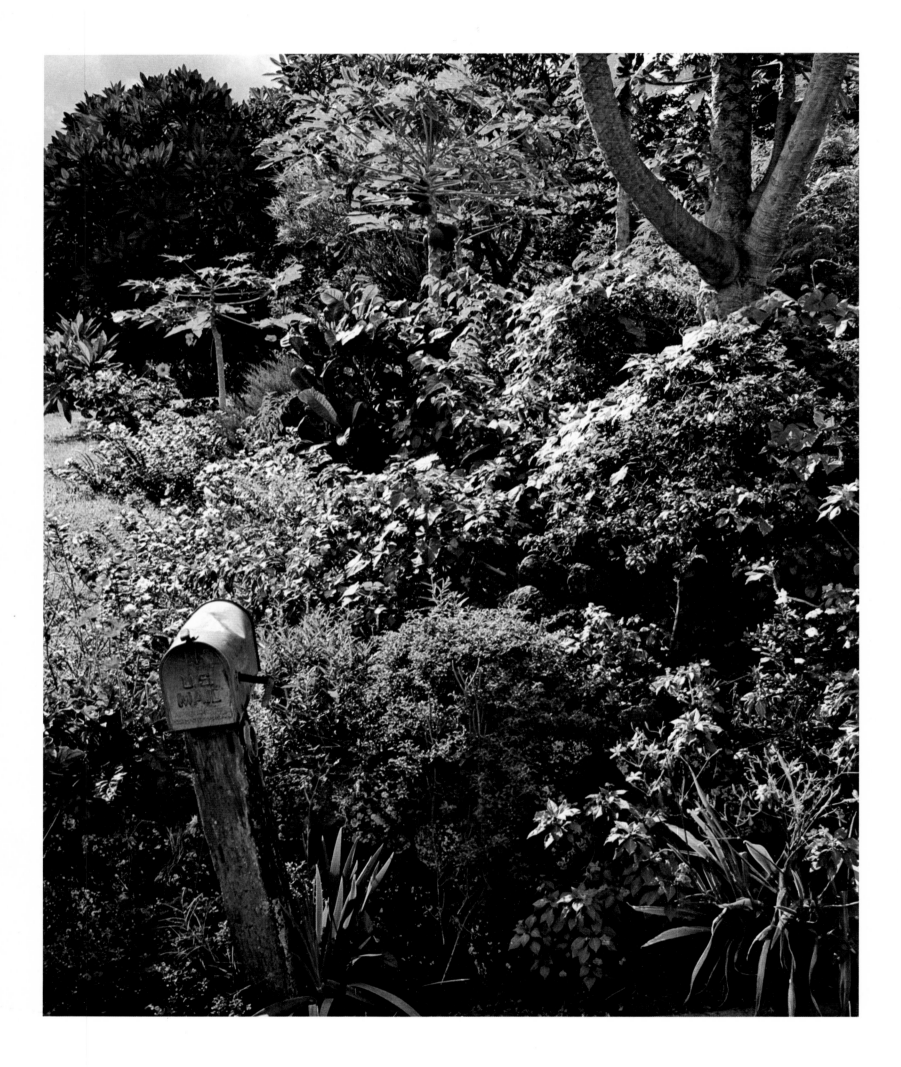

Herman Nelson

When Herman Nelson's foster mother, Mrs. Carolyn Kenui, heard Herman's name mentioned, her face lit up. Then she wrinkled her nose and made a little gesture of fond exasperation. "That rascal," she said.

Mrs. Kenui was sitting on the sofa in her living room, in the company of a daughter, two grandchildren, and her three visitors. She was a very old woman, so stooped, dry and light in the body that her hands and arms, dark brown against her light shift, seemed unnaturally large. Her hands were strong and gnarled, and were graceful as she absently stroked the toy bear of one of her grandchildren. Her hair still had much black in it, and was pulled back in a bun. She wore glasses with yellow-tinted, round plastic frames that looked like the old Army issue, and one lens was much thicker than the other.

Mrs. Kenui's house, painted green on the outside and lost in a profusion of broad tropical leaves, was small and neat inside. There were water stains on the ceiling, and some of the woodwork was warped with age and moisture,

but these were things that couldn't be helped. There was a sort of miniature altar in the middle of one wall. It had three plywood shelves that held tiny colored pictures of saints. There was a small cross on the middle shelf, carelessly hung with a lei of faded flowers. On either side of the altar were large oblong photographs on glass, one of a young Mrs. Kenui and the other of her young husband. The clothes they wear are very old-fashioned, and the Kenuis are expressionless, like the American Indians in photographs from the same period. The frames had been broken long ago, Mrs. Kenui told us. The glass had somehow survived. There were more recent, and smaller, photographs scattered over the other walls, as in all Kipahulu houses. There were wedding and graduation pictures, and portraits of children. One of the children on the wall, Herman Nelson's son, was present in the flesh—a handsome, shy, oriental-eyed boy seven years old who lay on the sofa near his grandmother and pretended not to listen to the conversation.

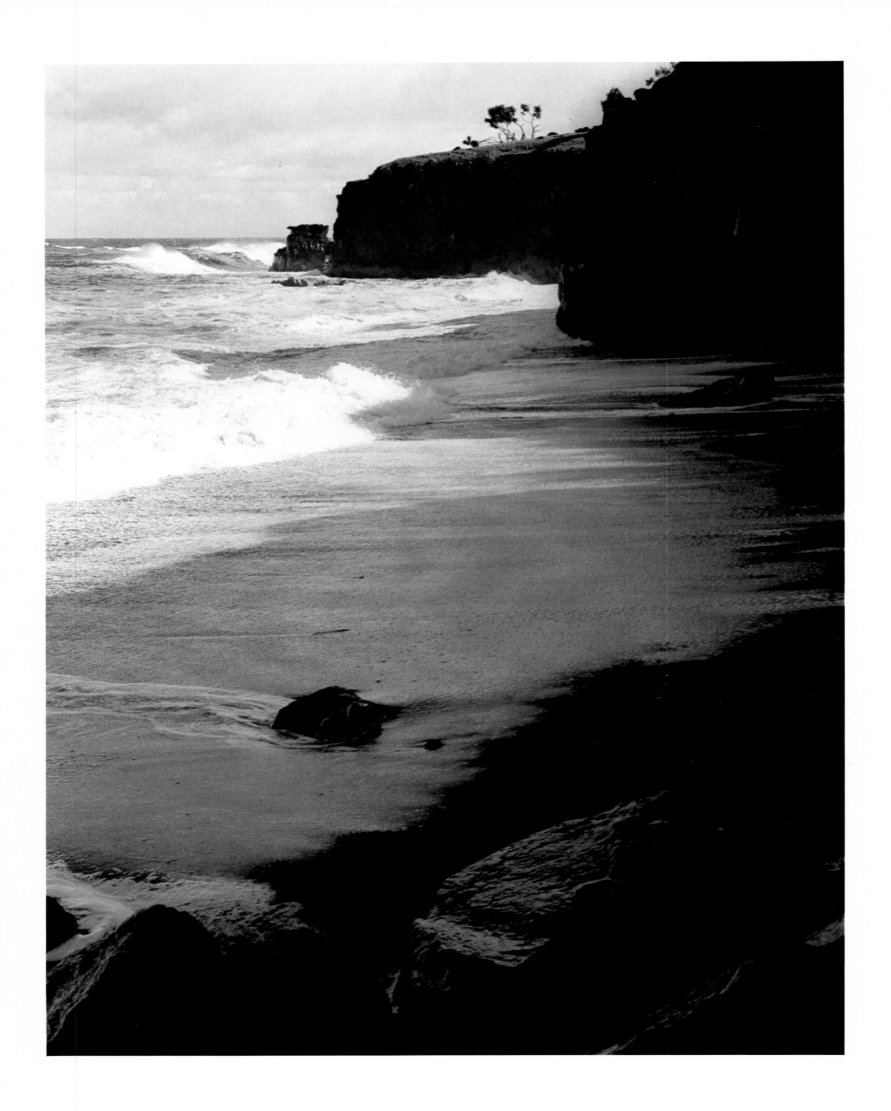

Mrs. Kenui's first language is Hawaiian, and her English is not good. As she talked about Herman, she often had to stop and search for the English word. She usually found it, and the story moved along well enough. She told about how her foster son made one of his early escapes from the house. He began by walking next door—an act that aroused no suspicion. Finding no one at home there, he turned on the neighbor's radio. Mrs. Kenui, hearing the radio, assumed that her neighbors were home and that Herman was playing there. It was only after a good while that she began to wonder why Herman had been gone so long and why the radio was playing so loudly. She went over and found the house empty. Herman had long since departed, on a donkey he had somehow acquired, had joined a young companion and was headed north.

Herman was always acting smart, Mrs. Kenui said, always pretending he knew more than you. She did not find this at all endearing, even now, looking back on it. She thought about the trait for a moment, stroking the stuffed bear, and then continued.

She told us how she got Herman back from Honolulu. He had worked there for a while as a young man, and she had worried about him, having heard of all the places there were in the city for a young man to get drunk. She knew that Herman liked a girl on his home island, and she engineered his return to Maui and his marriage there. Not until four children later did Herman get back, briefly, to Honolulu. It was a victory for Mrs. Kenui, and she still takes pride in it.

Mrs. Kenui spoke sadly of the state of Herman's mind. He could have been a good fisherman, she said. He had the kind of skill the old-time fishermen needed, in the days when they sighted distant schools of mackerel from high points of land and pursued them with boats and nets. Herman could have done it, she said, but he never put his mind to it. His mind wouldn't stick on things. She told him that he could make a little extra money for his family that way, but he never got around to it.

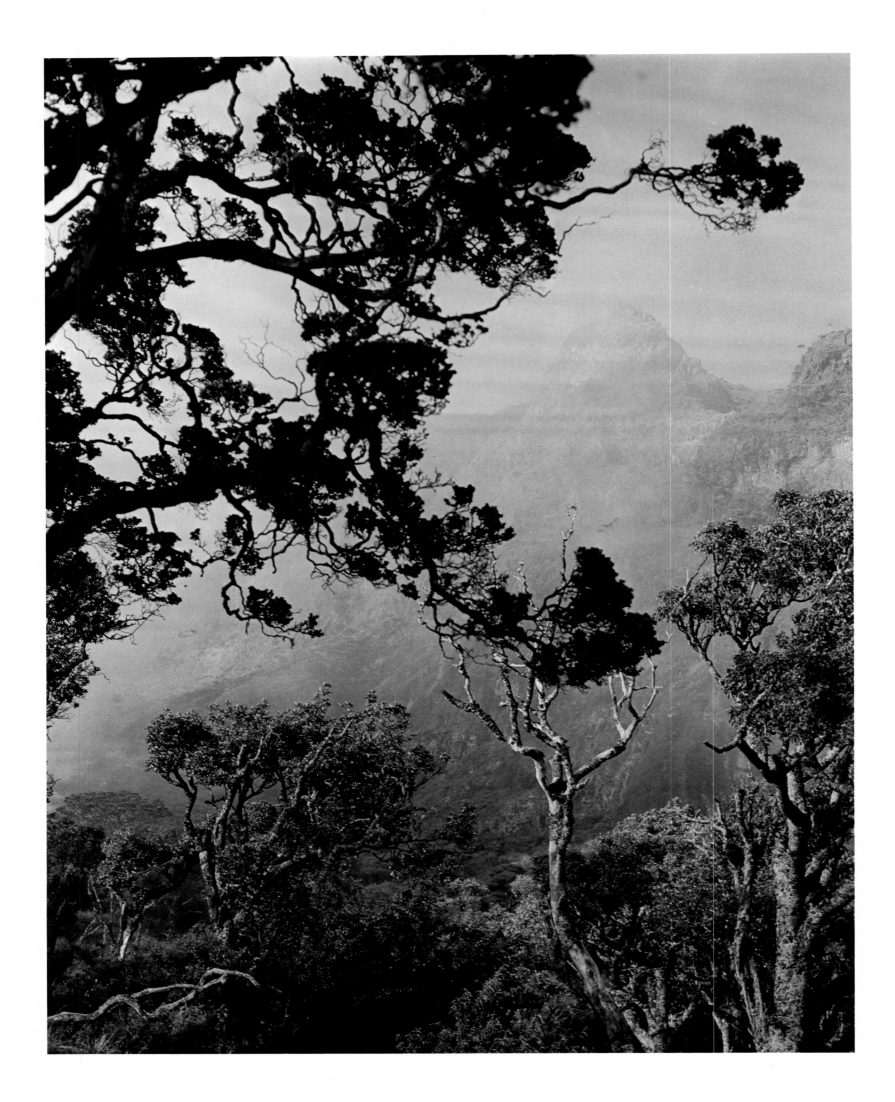

Herman Nelson's Hawaiian name is *Halemano*—House of the Shark. He is called *Mano* for short. Herman is a tall man, and when his shirt is buttoned to hide his substantial belly, he looks almost lean. His hair is always unkempt, as if he has just awakened, and he is never close-shaven, always stubbly, his beard a bit grizzled. He has heavy-lidded, smiling, sly yet good-natured, slightly Oriental eyes. He doesn't look at all respectable.

Herman supports his wife and nine children by working as a hand on the Kipahulu Cattle Company Ranch. On the ranch, and elsewhere in Kipahulu, he is considered the district's funniest and most interesting character. The people are modest about him, though. They know that Kipahulu is small and that Herman is probably not really a great character—that he wouldn't be famous in a big place where the competition was rougher. They are unsure of his stature as an anti-hero.

The feats that Herman's reputation is based on are not always sensational, it's true. But they are usually interesting. Herman can drink two cases of beer at a sitting, and has been known to drink from three bottles at the same time. His drinking manners are famous. For every bottle that he opens for himself, he opens one for you, and soon you are hopelessly behind him, a long line of open bottles before you. If Herman is drinking his beer from a glass, he'll pour one for you and offer it. If you refuse, he'll say, "come on man, or I'll drop it." If you refuse again, he'll let go of the glass, and as it shatters he'll begin pouring you another.

Herman's manners failed him once, at a party in Kaupo. He and some friends were drinking, passing around a gallon jug of wine. When Herman's turn came, he took the jug and climbed up a tree with it. He drank there at his leisure, while everyone below shouted at him to come down. After a while he did come down, not from good conscience or any return of his social sense, but because he slipped and fell the considerable distance to the ground. Everyone ran up, asking of the jug "Did it break? Did it break?" knowing enough about Herman not to worry about him, or not to care.

The Kipahulu people who tell this story know that its ending is predictable, and that the other drinking stories are somewhat homely. They are apologetic in telling them. They appreciate Herman, but don't expect others to. They make no great promises for him. "That Herman Nelson, he's a carefree fellah," is the most they'll say.

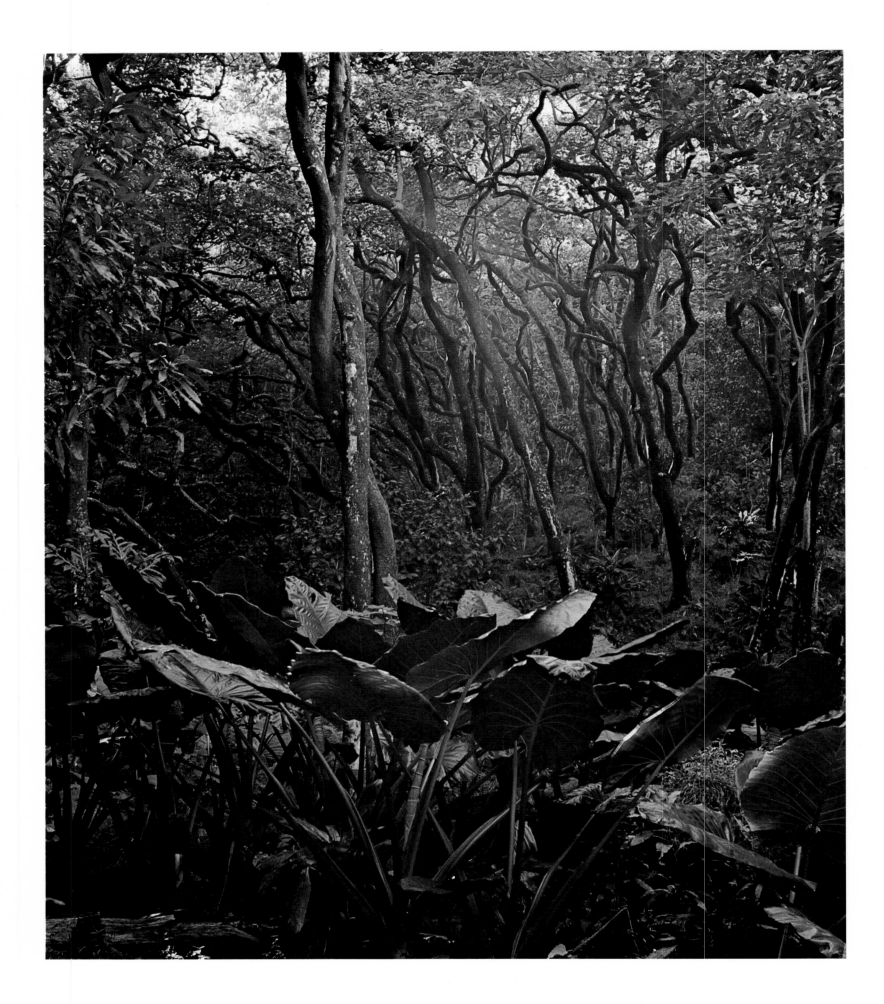

Jack Kaiwi, Herman's best friend, tells about the time Herman rode the wild boar. It happened one morning when Herman, Jack, and several friends were out hunting, following their dogs through the forest. The dogs picked up a boar's trail, gave chase, and caught him in a small clearing. They held him by the ears and waited for the men to come up.

When Herman saw how large the boar was, he had a thought, and said, "Jack, why don't we ride him?" Jack thought it was a good idea. (They were both a little high, Jack confesses—Herman as usual a little higher than Jack.) Herman got on in front as the dogs held the boar, and Jack got on behind. They shouted at the dogs to let go, and the boar took off.

Herman rode fairly easily, because his legs were so long that he could drag his feet on the ground. Jack's legs didn't reach, and his seat was more precarious. He had to lean with each of the boar's turns, like someone riding a motorcycle. He stayed on, though, and he was having a good-enough time. Then the boar caught sight of Herman's long legs behind him, and began turning tight circles on himself, trying to get at them. The ferns around the boar were leveled in circular swathes, and Jack noticed this. It was impressive testimony to the boar's determination, and Jack began to wonder if he and Herman hadn't made a mistake. Herman was having a good time and made no note of it.

The centrifugal force of the tightening circle finally threw Herman off, and the boar went for him on the ground. Herman kicked the boar away, and with Jack still riding, it took off again, the dogs in pursuit.

When Jack Kaiwi figured the time was right, he jumped off. He quickly looked back at Herman, and saw the blood running from his leg. Indignant at the boar for goring his best friend, Jack snatched up Herman's carbine. The dogs had prevented the boar from escaping, and Jack fired at him three times. "Missed that fellah!" Jack says, in recalling the incident today, and he is still bewildered that he could shoot so badly. The sights had been adjusted for Herman, and were no good for Jack. He tossed the carbine to Herman, and Herman shot the boar.

Herman was grinning as Jack walked back to him. He was too drunk to feel any pain. "Look at your leg, man," Jack said. "You're hurt." "Naaah," said Herman, but then he looked down at his leg.

Herman tried to get everyone to piss on it, but they couldn't, so he did it himself. Jack Kaiwi had no faith in this remedy, traditional and handy though it was. He found some guava shoots, applied them in a Hawaiian way, and slowed the bleeding. They carried Herman to the road and Herman's brother-in-law drove him to the hospital. The brother-in-law never exceeded the cautious fifteen miles per hour at which he always drives the narrow road to Hana. Herman passed out in the back seat from loss of blood. Jack Kaiwi, though he now remembers the boar fondly, is still indignant about the brother-in-law and the fifteen miles per hour.

Herman soon left the hospital, failed to return for his check-up, and his leg, which had been cut to the bone by the boar's tusk, infected. It smelled terrible, Jack confides, as he concludes his story, and in the end Herman had to spend three weeks in the hospital.

Ape leaves, kukui trees, Wailua Valley

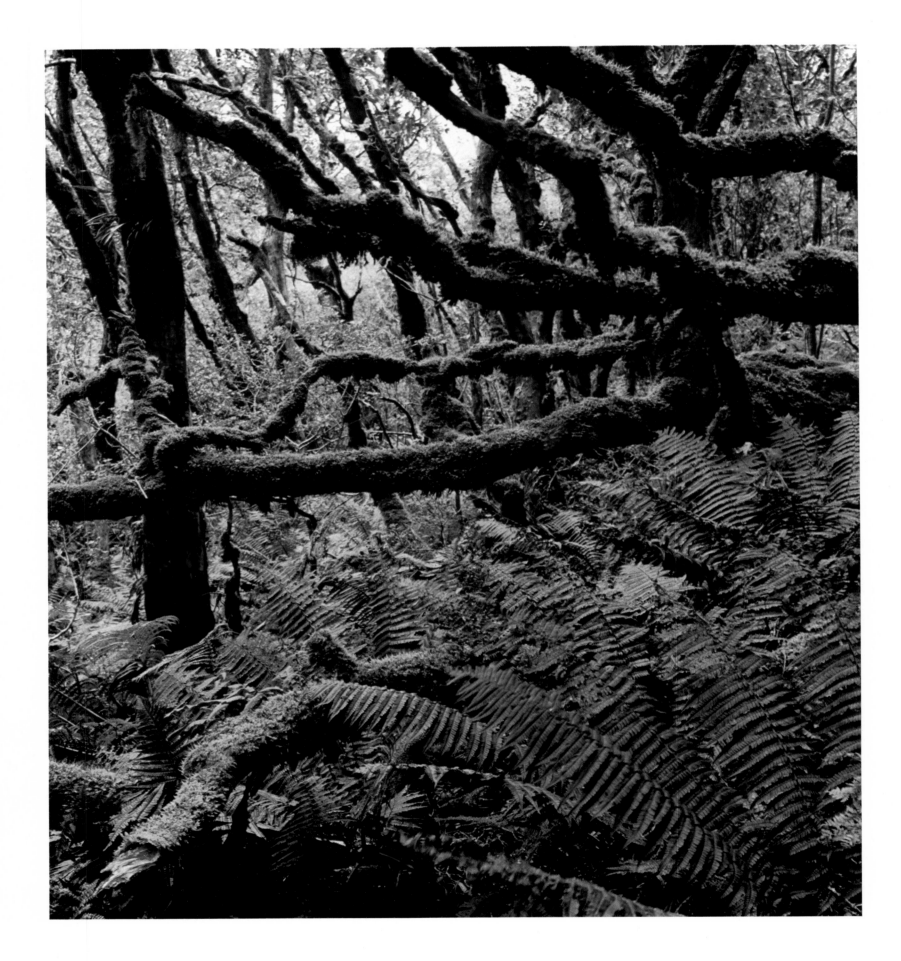

Another time Herman was hunting pigs in dense forest. He had two of them trapped in a gully, with no place to run except past him. He himself was restricted by the gully, unfortunately, and when the pigs rushed him he was standing with his legs spread, his feet against either gully wall. Herman was not perturbed, and as the first pig charged he swung his machete, killing it as it passed between his legs. The second pig was quicker, sadly, and Herman swung late, missing the pig and hitting his own leg. The wound took forty-two stitches to close, the great number testifying to the strength of both Herman's arm and his constitution. The doctor told Herman's friends that if he had not been a strong man, he would have bled to death. The friends were impressed. It's a rare man, they believe, who can inflict so much damage on himself and then recover from it.

Herman was sober the day of this accident, but he was drunk the night he hit the Black Angus bull and tore up the fender of his car. His excuse was that the bull was black and impossible to see. Herman was convincing in his amazement at how the animal got onto the road in the first place, and he stayed out of trouble. (The part about Herman's being drunk is supposed to be a secret, because Jack Lind, the ranch manager, doesn't know about it. It should be all right to tell it now, though, as the bull has since recovered.)

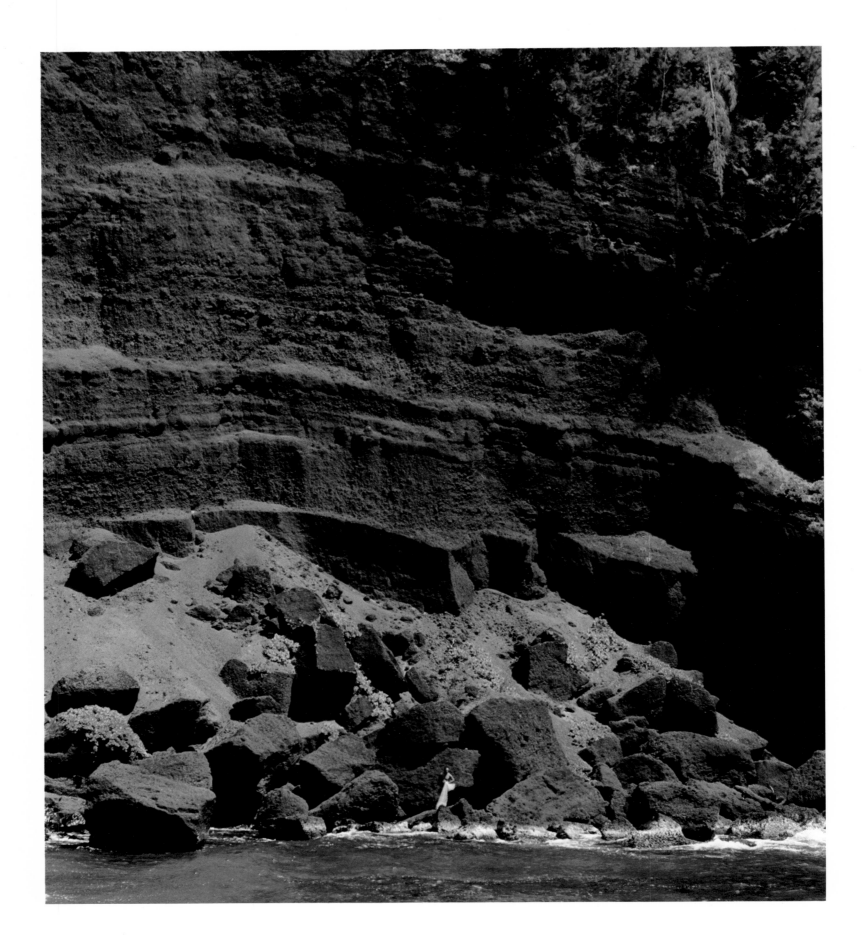

Herman's relations with the world are not all so abrasive. For every story about his recklessness, there is another about his gentler touch.

"This is where Herman Nelson comes to get *maile*," Paul Kaiwi told me one afternoon as we climbed the west ridge of Kipahulu Valley. Paul is Jack Kaiwi's oldest son, and has known Herman all his life. Paul bent a maile tendril in my direction to show me how the vine looked. Then he twisted it to loosen the epidermal sheath. He stripped the sheath off in one piece, as Herman had taught him, and put it in his sack. The maile smells faintly sweet when first picked, but after a few days drying in the house the sweetness fills the room. It is a favorite material for making leis.

The fragrance of beer is not, then, the only fragrance that moves Herman. If he is a rascal, as his mother said, he is not a standard rascal.

Later, as Paul Kaiwi and I returned through the guava forest, I noted the yellow guavas on the otherwise drab ground. Some of the fruit had been squashed in its fall, some partly eaten by pigs, with the pink insides showing. Each round guava was a minor world for a small population of fruit flies, which rose up as we passed. I asked Paul if anyone ever bothered to pick guavas. Herman Nelson did, Paul answered, but not most other people. Sometimes Herman took his whole family and some boxes and spent the day picking in the guava forest below the Hana road.

Herman is a diver and a fisherman, I learned later, as well as a hunter and gatherer. He enjoys being a man on an island. His skill at living off the land gives him a lot of pleasure—partly, perhaps, because it is a way to cheat his many creditors—but also because it is Hawaiian and sensible. He is at home in the Kipahulu country and deft in his relations with it, and this bit of sanity underlies all the raucousness of his public life.

Net fisherman, Ka'uiki Head

Surf, Keanae shore

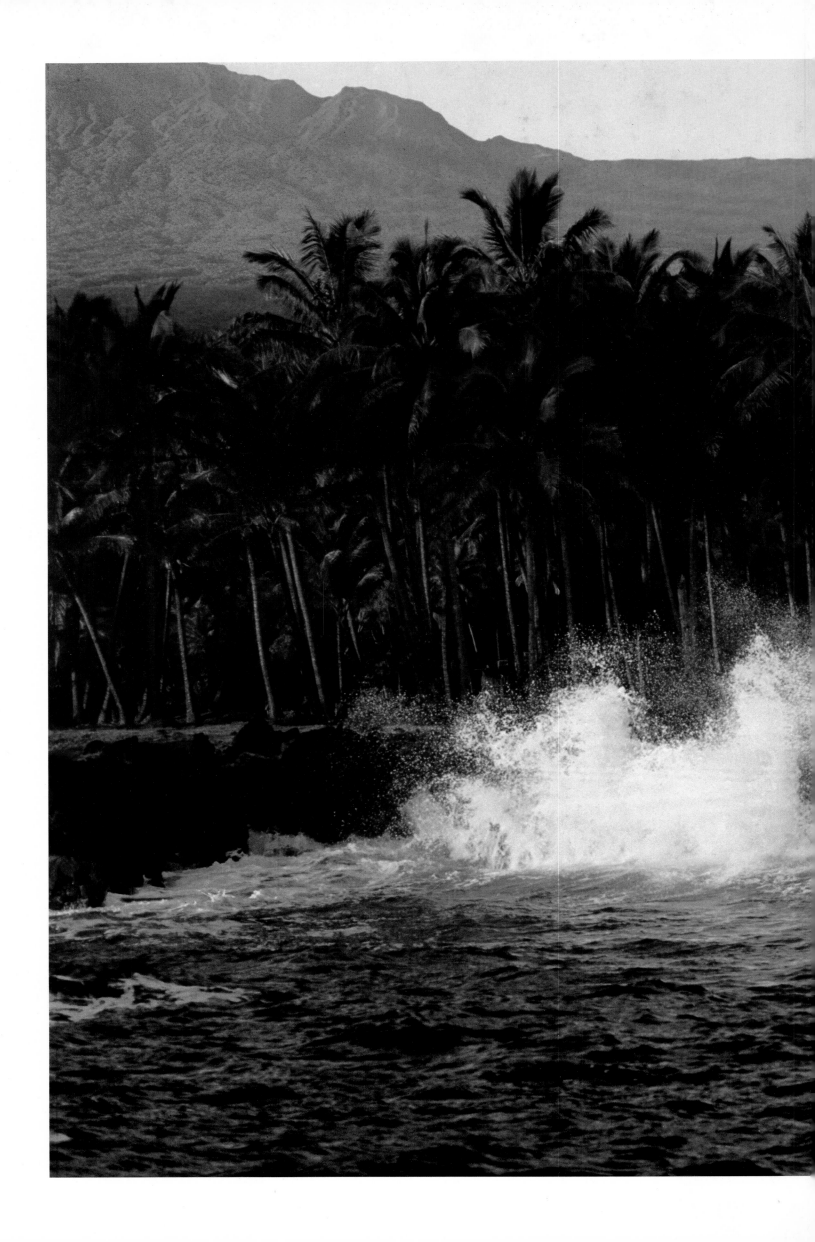

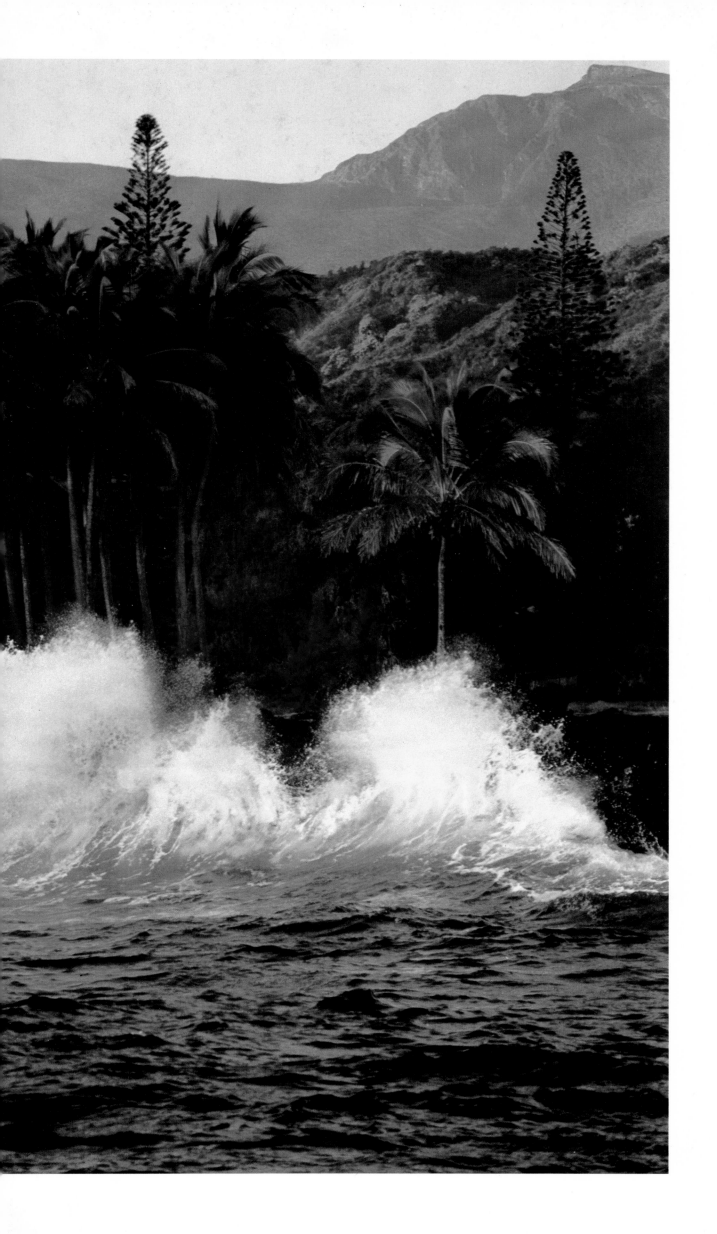

In Herman's gentleness and roguishness, in his two very different yet somehow not incongruous sides, he is very much like the demigod Maui, after whom his island is named. Maui had a kind of innocence. He was a fisherman and a kite-flyer, a player of string games, a solver of riddles, and sometimes a hero, as when he tried to kill Hina, the goddess of death. But he had a rascally side too. He turned his brother-in-law into a dog out of boredom, and set the world on fire by fooling with the fire goddess. He was responsible for giving the earth a reasonable amount of sunlight by crippling the sun and forcing it to traverse the sky more slowly, but he also starved his grandmother to obtain her magic jawbone. Maui was a lot like Coyote of Navajo myth, and a bit like Falstaff of Shakespearean myth. All three were good at bottom, but subject to frequent lapses of honesty, and each had a genius for getting into trouble.

Herman Nelson has a long scar on his right wrist, and little sensation in his hand. "Very nomb," as Jack Kaiwi says. The scar and the numbness are the result of an evening's drinking long ago in Honolulu. Herman was drunk, and his brothers, sitting in the car, teased him by rolling up the windows and making faces at him from inside. Herman punched at them, and his hand went through the glass. It was the kind of impulse Maui might have acted on, it seems to me, if he had been born in less heroic times.

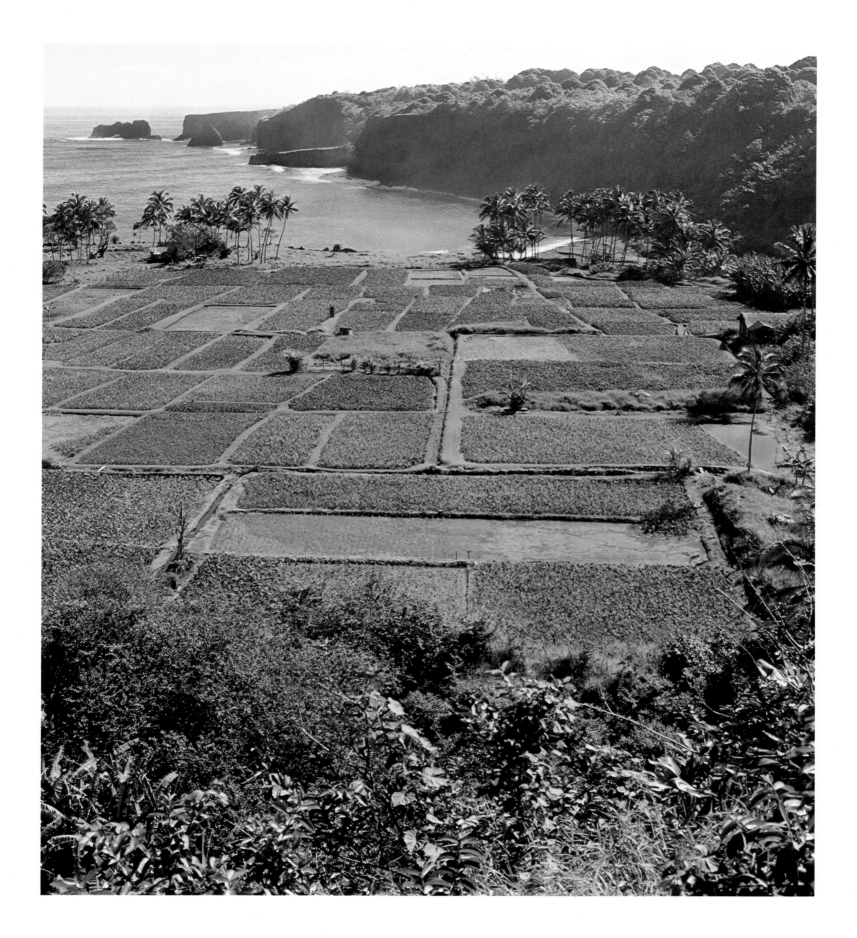

I was never able to check my opinion on Herman's resemblance to Maui with anyone on Maui's island, because no Hawaiian of Herman's generation had heard of the demigod. Mrs. Kenui may have known about Maui, but I forgot to ask her.

The demigod and the ranch hand may not be as much alike as I think. I learned about both men at the same time, and they have become somewhat confused in my mind. I walked around Kipahulu in the daytime, talking to people and hearing about Herman, and at night, by light of Coleman lantern, I read about Maui. It was hard for me to tell where one left off and the other began, except that Maui's powers were supernatural, and before his adventures began I had to light my lantern. Herman may in fact be less violent than Maui, and Maui a man of more curiosity than Herman. It does not seem so to me, however, and when I think of Maui I see him wearing Herman's face.

Unnamed falls, Kipahulu Valley

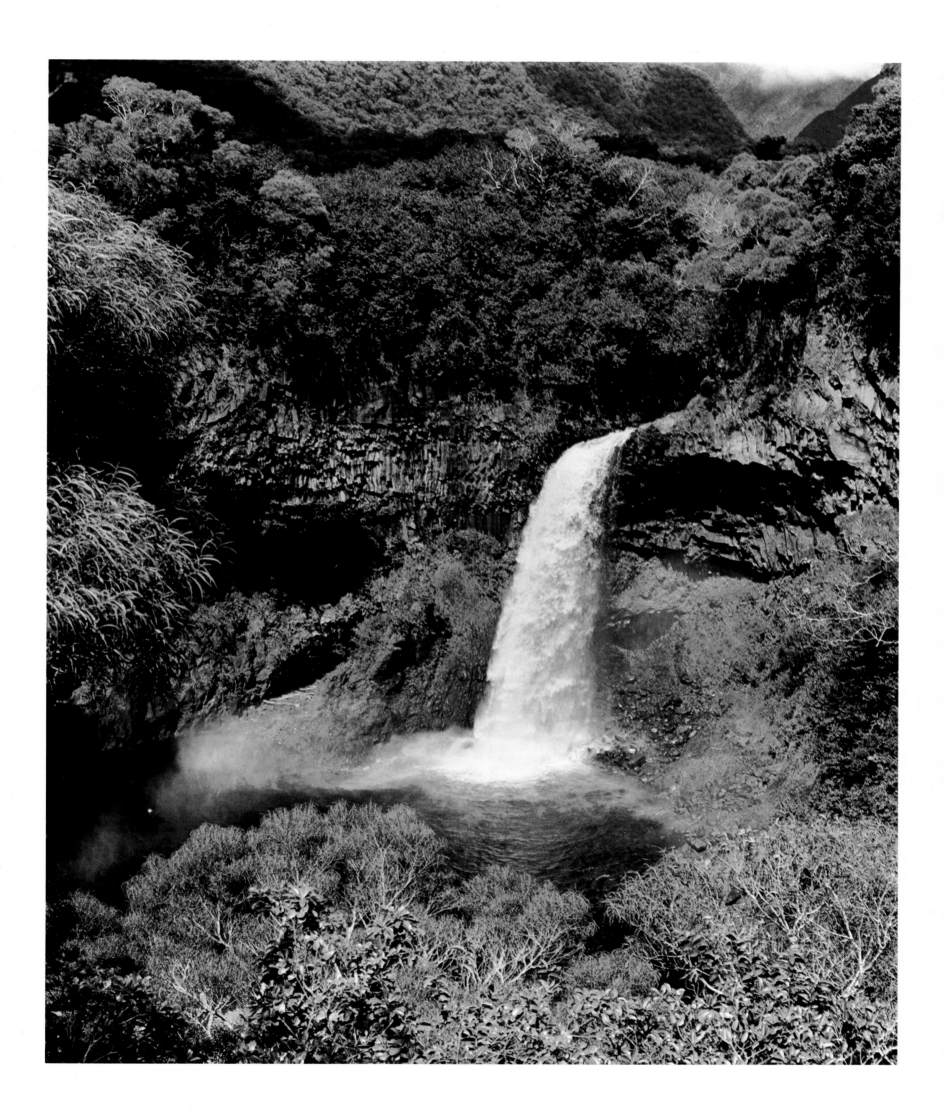

Visitors

Two flower children, driving their motorbike over the rough road from Kaupo, had reached Kipahulu when the bike broke down. The couple stood in the shade of a banana tree at the side of the road, thumbing for a ride into Hana. They had a long wait before a car came, for traffic in Kipahulu is light.

The boy was sturdy, had a short, sun-bleached blond beard and a reddish tan. He wore steel-rimmed spectacles and had a tattoo on his arm. He had the look of someone who has spent time in The Service before discovering the New Freedom. He still looked more naval than academic, in spite of the steel-rimmed glasses. The girl wore a swim suit and smiled continuously.

A car stopped, and they climbed in. They asked to be let off at Seven Pools. They were in no hurry to have the motorbike repaired. At the pools they would hitch another ride for the rest of the trip to Hana, and see about

fixing the bike later. They looked out the windows at the green country passing by them.

"Isn't this island out of sight?" the boy asked the driver. "Have you ever seen a place like this?" The girl said nothing, but continued to smile.

In Kipahulu, hippies are a new phenomenon. People like the couple above seldom come through, but those who do are objects of a mild curiosity. Kipahulu residents, when sitting together on front porches, speak disparagingly of hippies, but once alone everyone says he really doesn't mind them. No one feels threatened by the different way of life. Paul Kaiwi, for one, likes hippies well enough. When some of them walk down the road near where Paul waters the horses, he calls out to them.

"I have some water here. You want a drink?" They always accept, Paul says, and they always thank him.

Cinder cones, Haleakala

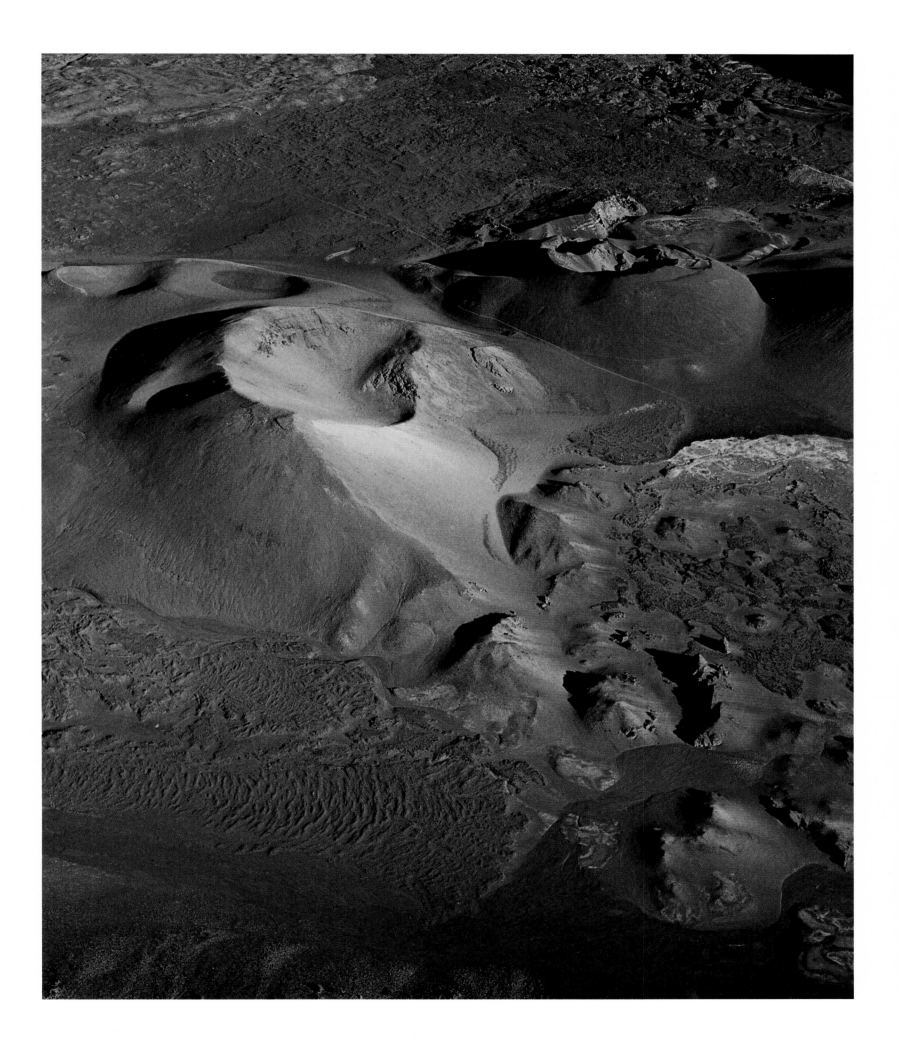

The Linds

Jack Lind has spent his life working on the land. He is a ranch manager now, but still has a ranch hand's forearms. The arms are tanned, as his face is, by the Hawaiian sun. He has short graying hair and mild blue eyes. The skin of his neck is seamed, as it often is in men of fair complexion who spend their lives under the sun. He looks fit, though like most men his age a little heavy in the midsection. Lind speaks clearly but quietly, with the diminished force of someone who has just run a race or put in a day's work. His voice is languid, but not weary; alert, satisfied, and at ease. It's the kind of voice you lean to hear.

The son of a Scot who settled in the Islands, Jack Lind has spent his life in his father's adopted country, and has been to the mainland only once. He has a slight accent— a touch of pidgin and perhaps a bit of his father's native brogue. He is a longtime cattleman, and the word "cattle-man" has an honorable, artisan sound in his mouth. He knows all the things you need to know in running a ranch. He can mend machinery, fences, and animals; he knows how to feed his stock, bargain for it, and ship it; he can please the ranch owner and get work out of the Hawaiian hands. He can shoe horses. He worries about web worm.

Lind is also one of those natives who are curious about their country. Most natives of a place become blind to it, but not all of them. Like Carmen Angermeyer of the Galápagos Islands, a fisherman's wife whose long observation of green turtles has proved valuable to marine biologists studying those creatures, and like Samuel Kamakau of the Hawaiian Islands, who recorded a great piece of his people's history before it vanished, Jack Lind is an islander who never ceased wondering. He is a shell collector and a birdwatcher. His pastimes might seem strange for a ranch foreman, but Jack is not embarrassed by them.

Old volcanic cone, Ulupalakua Ranch

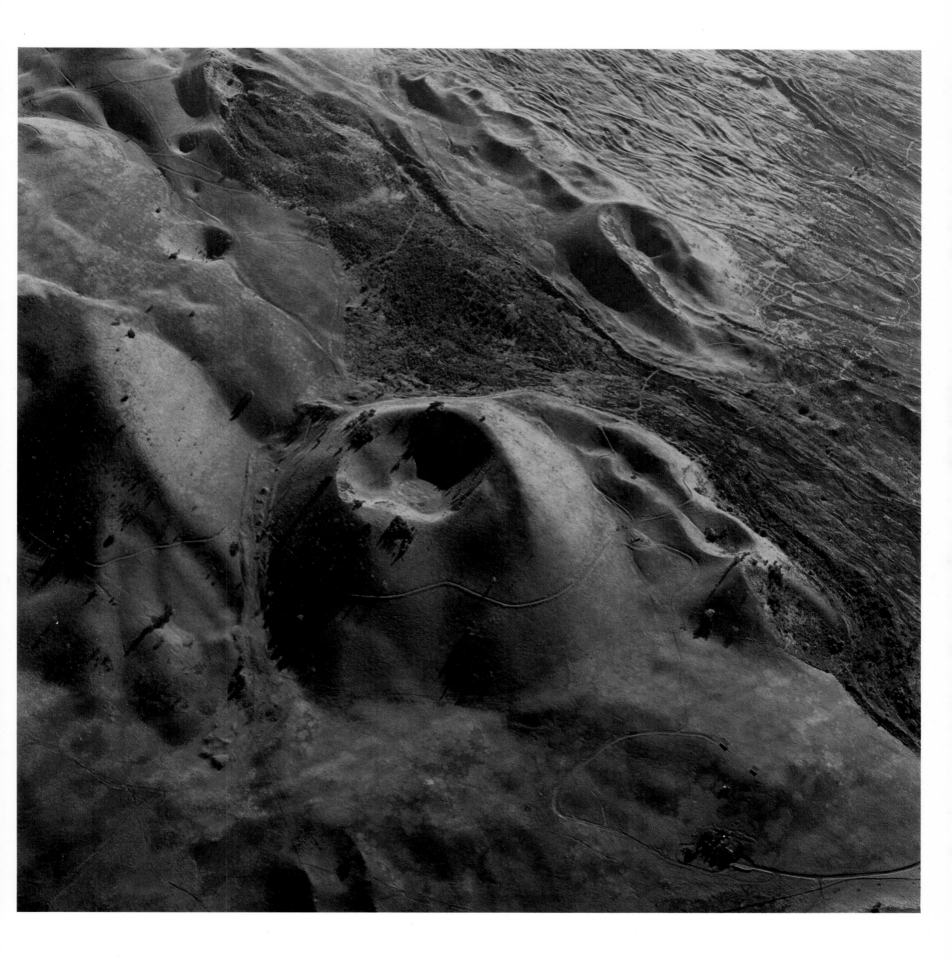

Jack Lind stood beside his Land Rover on a green hill near Seven Pools, waiting to take some visitors on a tour of the ranch. His Hawaiian wife Daisy sat in the back of the car and idly made something from flowers. She is a tallish, slender, pretty woman with beautiful hair, which on that day she wore in a pony tail. It is hard to believe, looking at her, that she has five sons and is a grandmother. You have to get close to see that her skin is not quite young. Jack stood by her, leaning easily with his elbow on her knee, and waited for his visitors to come up. After shaking hands, he went back to the knee. He made no effort to leave it, but leaned there lightly as he talked.

Daisy Lind is a bright and witty woman. Jack appreciates her, though she is noisier than he is, and her conversation is often more risqué than he would like. She has the old Hawaiian appreciation for jokes about sex. One afternoon, looking over nightgowns in a Wailuku store, Daisy fingered them indifferently and said, "The one I got at home, I wear it, I don't go to sleep all night." On occasions like this Jack looks at her in amazement, and looks around in an embarrassed way to see how many heard it, but he can seldom help but smile.

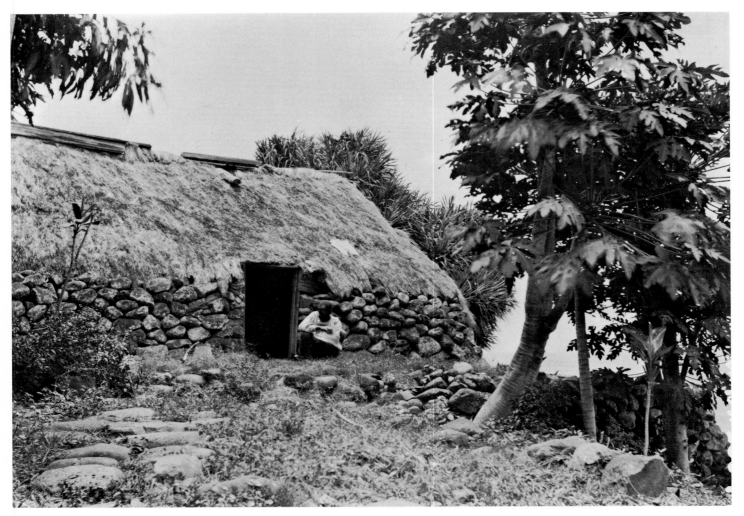

Grass hut, Kipahulu shore (about 1909)

At night Daisy Lind works as a bartender at the Hana hotel. She wears full Hawaiian gowns and arranges her hair beautifully on the top of her head. When business is slow, she sits behind the bar and works on her leis. In the daytime Daisy visits her neighbors. The trips she makes around Kipahulu in the family car or one of the ranch Land Rovers are the threads that tie the female society of the district together. She is likely to turn up, in an afternoon, on any of the nine or ten family porches of Kipahulu. She is the First Lady of Kipahulu, a lady in the unselfconscious tradition of Ka-ahumanu, the great, barefoot Hawaiian queen who so impressed the Russian explorer Kotzebue, in spite of himself, with her raw queenliness. When Daisy says "Pardon my French," it sounds clever and urbane.

Visiting old Mrs. Kenui, Daisy is her most open. She and Mrs. Kenui are among the last who speak Hawaiian, and they talk and laugh in that language. Daisy teases Mrs. Kenui about getting a new husband. Mrs. Kenui, a widow, grimaces and says she doesn't want another husband. The one she had, he came home late when she was asleep, and it was always tickle, tickle, tickle. Daisy laughs hard. If she has heard the story before, she pretends not to have.

Visiting Annie Smith, Daisy is more dignified. Annie Smith is a landowner and has a conservative air about her. The sign outside her small home reads "Mr. and Mrs. Louis Smith." Inside, the gay colors of her sofa, the white walls, the matting on the floor, would please the editor of any magazine of western living. Only two items would not please him: one, a tall felt cat in the Walt Disney tradition; the other a large tapestry showing two polar bears on an iceberg in a red arctic ocean under a red arctic sky. The polar scene might have a cooling effect, in Mrs. Smith's warm Hawaiian living room, if the dominant color were something different. The rich red the artist picked makes a summer visitor vaguely uncomfortable.

Daisy and Helene Kaiwi were visiting Mrs. Smith one morning. The women first talked about the hippies whose motorbike had broken down near the Smith's house. The hippies had entered the house—in Kipahulu no one has locks on his doors—and had used the telephone and bathroom. Mrs. Smith was offended, and Helene Kaiwi seemed to sympathize with her. Daisy reserved judgment.

The women talked on. They spoke, without ever properly gossiping as mainland women might, about a wealthy lady who vacationed in Hana. They talked about Hawaiian racial mixtures. Daisy told her friends about a mixed couple, Negro and White, that she had seen in a department store in Wailuku. The couple's child was very dark, almost black, with blond hair. Daisy's listeners both *aaahed* at this. They thought it must have been very striking and beautiful, and Daisy assured them that it had been. The women sat for a moment imagining it—Daisy remembering it—then they resumed the conversation, which became a bit freer. Daisy told about the time she knocked her uncle down. He was a big man who had been living in New York for fifty-three years. He came home and began saying that Maui was a pigsty. "The mainland makes this place look like nothing," he said, and he continued on that note until Daisy knocked him down. She swung again, but missed the uncle and hit the wall, cutting her knuckle. She showed everyone the small scar.

There are more than seventy miles of road between the ranch and Wailuku, where Daisy does her shopping, but she knows most of the cars she passes on the way. She and the occupants smile, wave, and exchange gay greetings. One large Hawaiian driving a truck grins broadly from his cab. Daisy fought him once, when they were young, over the price of coconuts. The Hana schoolchildren used to sell drinking coconuts to each other for a quarter. The truckdriver had taken her coconut and only given her a nickel. She had pursued him, given battle, and won. Now she waves at him as he passes.

Daisy takes off her headband and shakes out her long hair. The wind from the open window blows the hair out behind her. A car full of tourists passes. "Hey bruddah!" Daisy shouts in pidgin for their benefit, and waves gaily. One tourist, a man, waves freely back. The others wave uncertainly, not sure whether the Hawaiian woman with long hair streaming is making fun of them.

Daisy turns on the radio. She likes country and western music, but before she can reach the selector she hears "Hasegawa General Store," and she turns the volume up. The Hasegawa Store song, which almost made Hana famous, is a singing grocery list. It simply describes all the things you can buy at Hasegawa General Store—a truly amazing variety of items. Daisy must have heard it hundreds of times, but she listens again.

Daisy drives very fast. As she passes the grassy driveways of relatives and friends, she toots her horn, even when no one is in sight. Perhaps the friends look out the window in time to see Daisy disappear, or perhaps they know from the sound of the horn that Daisy has just passed by.

The Linds live in a forty-foot trailer that overlooks the Pacific. Their front door opens on the ocean, their back door on the high, green, cloud-capped slopes of Hale-akala. The trailer is set in the middle of pastureland, and the large yard is fenced against the cattle. A small addition has been built next to the trailer, and in it sleep the three Lind sons who have yet to leave home.

The inside of the trailer is crowded and sometimes a bit messy. The Linds are not an orderly family, and if they did not spend most of their time outside, the trailer would surely be impossible to live in. Both Daisy and Jack have a feeling for objects and have filled the trailer with them. Hawaiians are still flower people, and Daisy's flowers are everywhere. Coke bottles, ballasted with different kinds of sand, serve her as vases, and they line the walls. Most of the flowers are real, but some are artificial. On her shopping trips to Wailuku Daisy spends much of her time in the shops where ideas for making flowers are on display. There is a great range of colors, textures, shapes, and possibilities, all aimed at female Hawaiian shoppers faithful to their ancestry. Daisy's own flowers are bright and tasteful inventions, few of them resembling any species known to man, but all of them following infallibly the principle of a flower, the design guided by the instinct of the race whose understanding of flowers is deepest.

Above Daisy's sofa are graduation photographs of her two oldest sons—one works in Honolulu, the other is away at war. The photographs are draped with yellow leis.

Jack's shells fill a glass case that stands behind the kitchen table. Some of the shells are rare for Hawaii, some rare for any place, yet Jack hands them to you impartially, and is not solicitous about them. Diving for them is the important part for him, apparently. On a small table is a piece of hardwood Jack brought down from Kipahulu Valley. It is planed and polished on one side, with "Kipahulu Valley Expedition 1967" burned into the smooth surface. The wood is iron hard, and it caused the expedition, which Jack helped organize, considerable difficulty when they tried to cut through it.

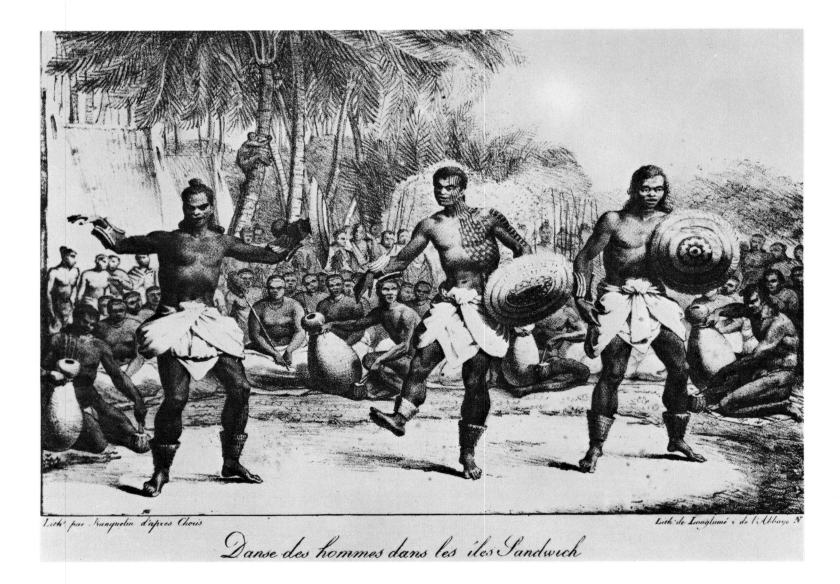

Lith. par Franquelin d'après Choris   Lith. de Langlumé : de l'Abbaye N.

Danse des hommes dans les îles Sandwich

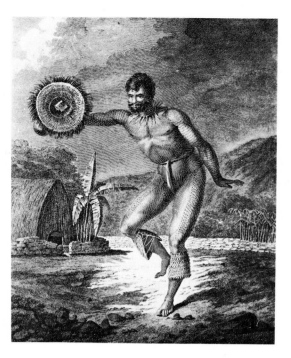

Dinner at the Linds has been a somber occasion of late. The boys don't get out of wrestling practice until nine in the evening, and it takes them half an hour to drive home. Their parents are alone in a quiet trailer until then. They are getting a taste of what life soon will be like when their youngest son, now fifteen, leaves home. They have decided they don't like it.

Daisy fixes Jack a plate; some rice and fried fish caught by one of her uncles. She pours him a glass of passionfruit-orange nectar, and sets on the table a bowl of opihi shellfish, collected the day before by one of her sons who, shirtless and wet, cut them from the rocks below the Lind's promontory, turning his face away each time the surf broke over him, putting the opihis in the sack at his waist. Later Daisy fixes a plate for herself.

There is nothing festive about Daisy's table. The passion-orange nectar is Haleakala brand, with a picture of a silversword on the carton, but this is accidental decoration and otherwise things are dull. The two parents eat without much spirit, and watch television or read until the boys come in.

The boys enter sweating and shirtless. They left the gymnasium that way—or two of them did, the third wearing a wet T-shirt—but the night air is warm and they do not catch cold. The oldest son has just driven over the dark stretch of road he has driven so many times before, his two perspiring brothers and he filling the Volkswagen, his headlights picking up African toads on the wet road, toads that he avoids by minor corrections of his wheel. There can't be much pleasure in driving the road one more time, and it must be good to turn off at the home gate.

The nightly Lind reunion is not especially noisy or gay. Of the Lind sons, only the youngest is at all talkative. The older two are quiet, and rarely speak to their parents un-less spoken to. There is nothing sullen about their silence, but simply little eagerness for talk. The arrival of the boys changes the trailer, though. There is an awakening. When the thin hunting dogs on the front step raise their ears and then their heads, and turn them toward the distant sound of the Volkswagen, there is a quickening about the trailer, an imminence, and the Linds become a family again.

The boys must be grateful for the quiet of the trailer. The small bungalow that serves as a gym for Hana wrestlers is crowded and chaotic, and the Lind sons spend three hours a night in it. There are wrestlers of all ages and sizes, the smallest of them awkward in outsized wrestling suits and often not very serious about their sport. It must be a difficult place for a dedicated athlete to practice his art. The Linds are dedicated, especially Greg, the oldest, whose trophy for having been Maui's outstanding wrestler stands with his father's shells. The Lind's Hana team was badly defeated last season by a more experienced team from Honolulu, and there is a grimness to this season's preparations. After three hours of concentration and effort, food and rest must be good.

After they eat, the Lind sons, still shirtless, join their mother on the sofa and watch television. Duffy sits with a leg sprawled over his mother's. His mother leans an elbow on Greg's knee, puts her chin in her hand, and from this vantage regards the screen. If Greg is annoyed by the contact, or even notices it, it is not apparent from his eyes, which, weary and no longer very alert, stay on the T.V.

The Linds, like other Hawaiian families in Kipahulu, are not particular about the privacy of their persons. They have an easy intimacy uncommon on the mainland. In Kipahulu, it seems, you are not so aware of where your own body leaves off. The Lind family, on wrestling nights at least, is one body.

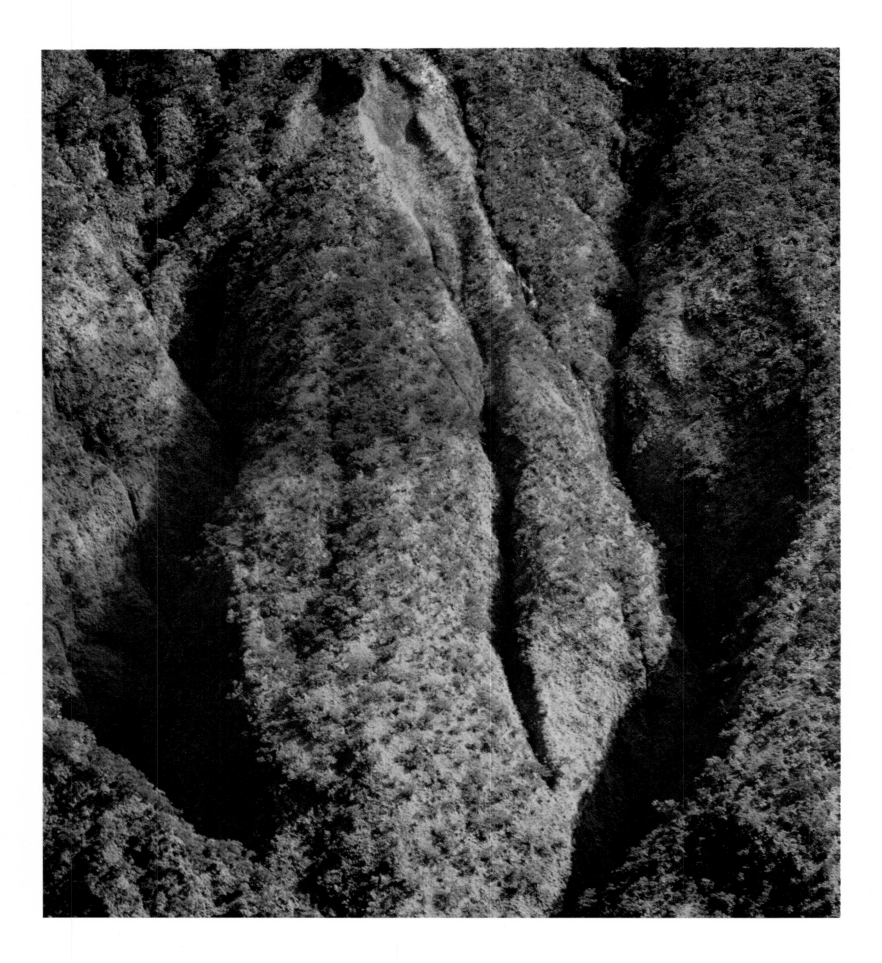

One clear November morning Jack Lind and I walked up the west ridge of Kipahulu Valley. We had driven a jeep to the edge of the high pasture, parked, and entered the guava forest on foot. We climbed for a while through guava trees, with fallen fruit and a dry litter of leaves under foot, until the guavas gave out and the native forest of koas and pulu ferns began. We climbed through the koas until we came to where the ohia forest started, and there we made camp.

Walking on the razorbacked ridgetops was easy. The high spine of the ridge was so sharp that it held no water, and the forest there was not thick. These ridgetops are the only ways to get back into the country. The forest of the valley bottom is impenetrable, the mud there knee deep, and the precipitous walls of the valley's ridges are slippery and tortuous; but the very tops of the ridges, sometimes only two yards wide, are natural trails to the center of the island. There is a satisfaction in looking back at Kipahulu's west ridge, and the other ridges of East Maui once you have tried them, and knowing about the secret and unlikely routes up.

The high Maui jungle is pleasant to look at as you walk. The forest is not so tangled that the eye has trouble organizing it. There are clearings here and there of a low, softer green, and their negative space is restful. There is a plant with leaves like elephant ears—leaves large enough to delineate themselves against their green backgrounds. These, and the rounded, whitish, rolling forms of kukui trees descending the ridges, give shape to what might otherwise be an amorphous exuberance of growing things.

Cliff, Kipahulu Valley

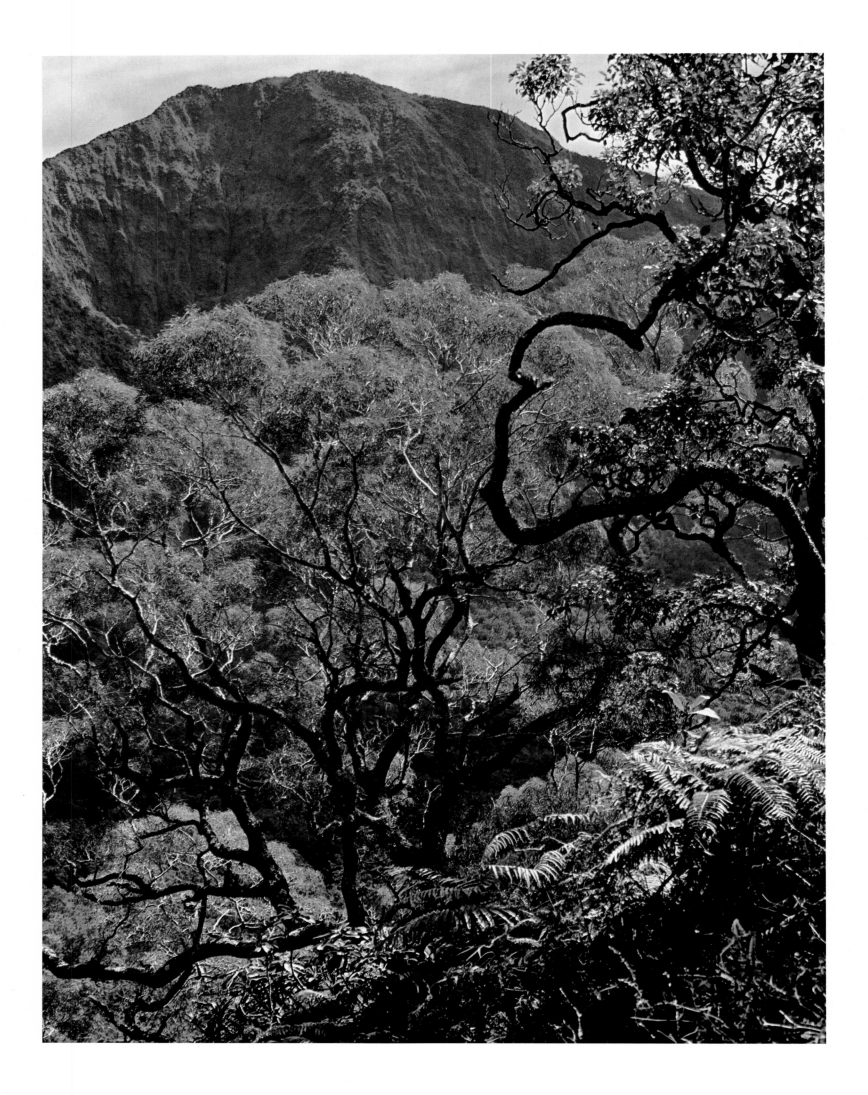

Our camp was in a clearing on the ridge just large enough for our two tents. Jack had camped here before, and he looked about with satisfaction. In season this jungle was red with ohia blossoms, he told me. The blossoms were sparse now, but Jack hoped that a few birds would be attracted to the ohias anyway.

Jack was carrying a camera and a telephoto lens. He had bought them after the Kipahulu Valley expedition of 1967. Jack, the *sirdar* of the expedition, had heard that the scientists were interested in rare birds of the valley, and had told them that he had seen nukupuu there. No one believed him. When an ornithologist on the expedition finally did see a nukupuu, the ornithologist reported it as the first seen on Maui since 1896. The bird had been discovered. It annoyed Jack not to be believed, and he bought the camera and lens. He has seen a bird that has yet to be discovered on the island of Maui, and he is ready for its next appearance.

We rested from our climb, and Jack told me about a botanist from the Pacific Botanical Gardens who had come up here. He had told Jack about prefabricated aluminum houses that you can buy in Japan. You can bring them to places like this, the botanist said, assemble them, and live in them while you cultivate gardens of rare flowers, small gardens fenced with hogwire against wild pigs. Little is known about the flowers of these ridges, and close study will be necessary if botanists are to know more.

Jack pointed out the place he felt was best for the house. "I wouldn't mind living up here, tending a garden," Jack said, as an afterthought.

I realized suddenly how differently Jack and I saw this country. The high Kipahulu jungle was a nice place to visit, I had thought, but who would want to stay here long? What kind of man would need, or desire, this kind of solitude? The Kipahulu jungle was a pleasant, but inhuman place. Two *iiwis* were calling from the forest.

Their calls sounded like a door creaking to Jack, and like electronic music to me. It was not the kind of sound that most men would want to wake or sleep to. And even at that, the iiwis and the other birds of the ridge were more vocal than visible. They stayed in the trees and were poor companions. The real king of the place was a large blue dragonfly who with a papery whirr of wings moved precisely through the tangled green. The dragonfly, and the tropical plants strange to me, made the ridge seem a ridge of another age—Mississippian or Pennsylvanian perhaps, and not right for a warm-blooded creature.

I wondered how this forest of koa and ohia looked to Jack; what it was he saw here that I did not see. I asked him if he really meant what he said about living here, and he said sure. It was clear that he had dreamed about it.

After a lifetime of work under the Hawaiian sun, on rolling pastures skimmed by plover, a life out in the weather, mending fences and looking after cattle, Jack was considering this ridge as a retiring place. For a man of curiosity who had lived a pastoral life, a house in Honolulu would have seemed more likely. Instead he was thinking of simply going up the hill, several thousand feet above his old pastures, pastures that he would see on a clear day from his aluminum station.

The pretty wife on whose knee he had leaned so easily, the five strong sons, the ranch he ran, the friendly Hawaiian homes where he was known and welcome, did not satisfy everything that needed satisfaction in him, apparently. He was considering a solitary perch in almost constant cloud and frequent rain, in wet forest where the iiwi calls and the nukupuu still lives. Whether it was the frustrated scientist in him, looking forward to the study of rare flowers after too much mending fence, or whether it was something else, is hard to say. Jack Lind must be a very peaceful man, though, to contemplate with equanimity all that simplicity and peace.

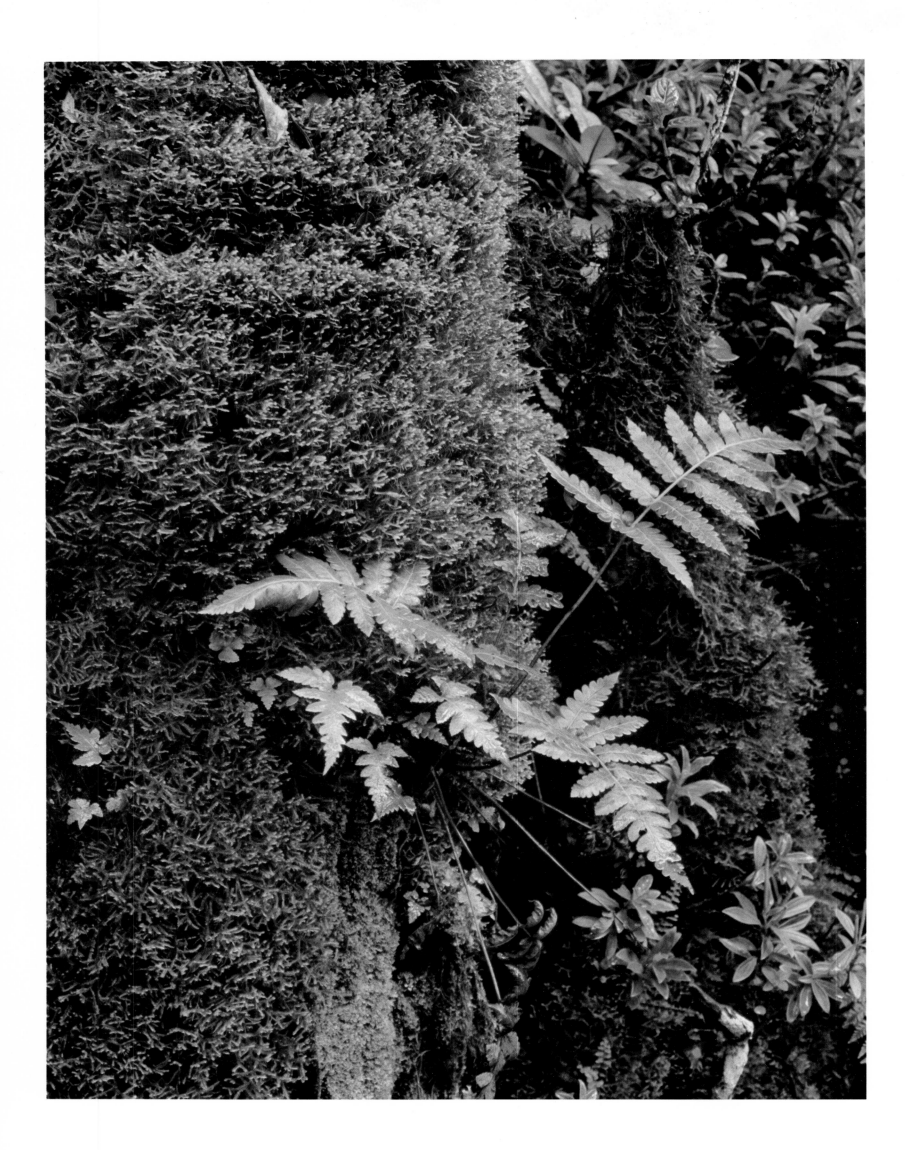

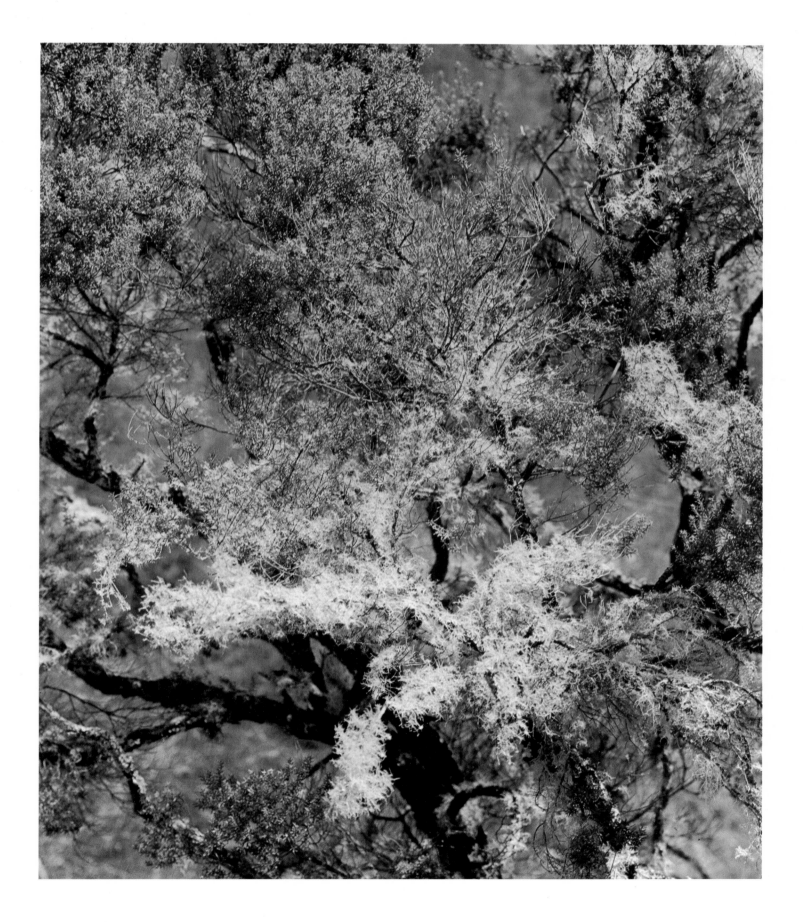

The sky was clear when we went to our tents that evening, but shortly after dark the wind came up and it started to rain. It rained all night, and by early morning nothing in our tents was dry. A seventy-mile wind blew out of the valley. We were in the lee of the ridge and partly protected, but our tents were still buffeted. Each time my tent snapped, the little lake at my feet splashed, and I don't remember sleeping. When we got up after dawn, we looked across and saw the far wall of the valley running white with hundreds of waterfalls.

It continued to rain, and we decided if we were to get dry, we would have to go down. We cached our food where the pigs couldn't get it, and started down the ridge.

The jungle was beautiful in the rain. The country was most intimate when rain and mist closed it in. As visibility decreased, near things jumped out at us. Greens became prettier in the subtler light. And when we were thoroughly wet, we ceased to mind the rain. Once as wet as the leaves, we could move through them carelessly. We were part of the country in a way we weren't before our own surfaces and the green surfaces around us shared a common shiny wetness.

As I pushed my way through fronds and ducked under a low branch, I happened to look at my shoulder and saw a delicate gray slug there. It was not likely that the slug had mistaken me for a leaf and deliberately crawled onto me, for slugs crawl slowly and I was moving fast, but I appreciated his gesture nonetheless. I had almost certainly brushed him off roughly in my passage under his leaf, but he had found my shoulder a cool and moist-enough substitute. His feelers were extended to their limits and he gave every other mollusk sign of comfort and confidence. As I had probably carried him for some distance already, I put him down, on a real leaf, and walked on.

When the Maui rain fell too hard, there were trees to stop under. The lee of a tree is the best place from which to watch a forest under rain. Watching rain, from the protection of tree or cave, is an older human habit than watching fire, and just as hypnotic. Jack and I stopped when the rain became too refreshing, and, waiting for it to let up, we watched it fall. The Kipahulu forest came alive as it received the rain. Each narrow blade and broad leaf danced as the rain struck. The raindrops followed each other closely down. The world became particled. The falling raindrops seemed, in shape and number, incarnations of the leaves. Our descent was slippery, but cool in the rain, and quick. We left the ohias behind, and passed through the koa forest, where several of the larger trees had cracked or fallen in the last night's wind. We left the koas behind, passed quickly through the guava forest, and came out in open pasture.

I reached the jeep first, and waited for Jack to arrive. I sat in the jeep, and watched the angle of the rain against the vertical lines of the guavas that bordered the pasture. The close-cropped grass danced all around me as the rain hit. As I watched, small pools formed in the grass. In places where the pools lay in a line, there were shortly small rivulets connecting them. The rivulets were at first only a fraction of an inch deep, but they ran fast, and tufts of grass kicked the water up into tiny rapids. Below, the rivulets became streams, and the streams rivers. The rivers were minor Colorados, running red and silty. The hills roared to the great volume of water running off them, and the surrounding sea, for hundreds of yards out, was brown with soil that had washed away.

Jack came up. He held in either hand a plant he couldn't identify. He planned to send them to a botanist friend, he said, and told me that he had slipped and fallen twenty times in trying to descend the ridge, encumbered as he was, without using his hands. His yellow "Kaapu for Mayor" T-shirt was wet through, his pants were muddy, and rainwater was running off his nose and chin, but he was smiling.

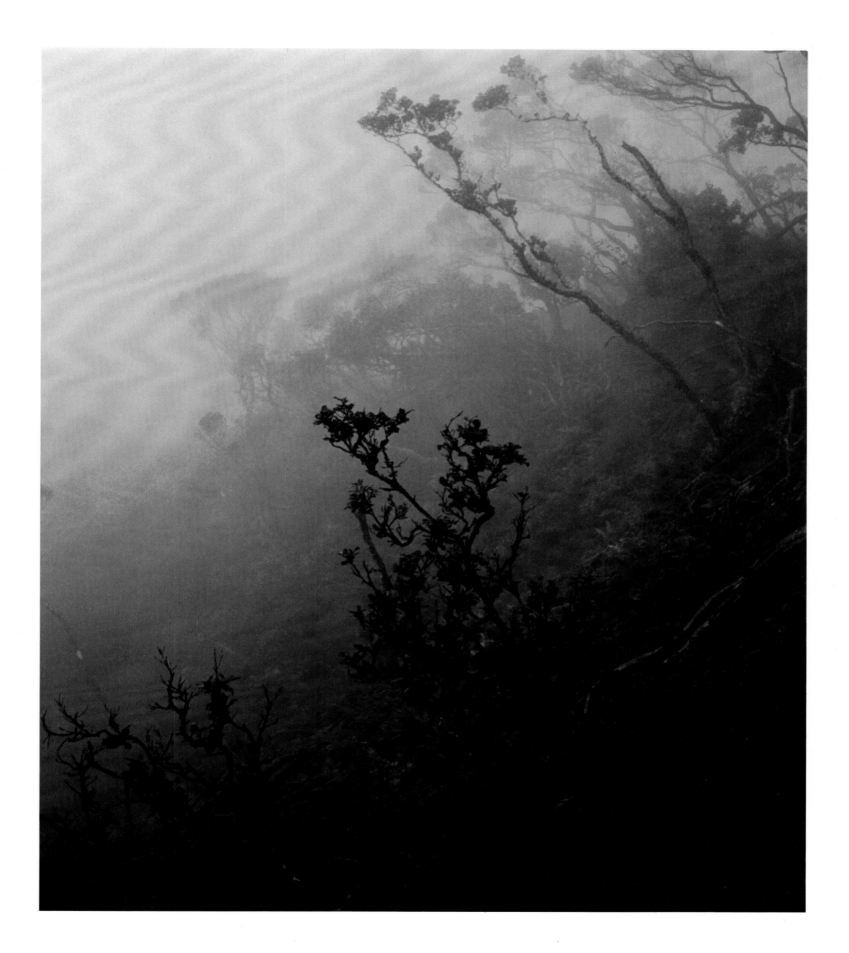

William Rost

William Rost, driving home from Hana, stopped and gave me a lift. I did not look closely at him as I got in. I did notice that his wife was Hawaiian, that the grandchild in the seat beside him was the old-ivory color of most Hawaiian babies. I noticed that though Rost's own skin was brown, his features were Caucasion and his eyes very blue. A white man. Then he spoke, in a pidgin as thick as any I had heard, and I leaned forward in my seat to have a closer look at him.

A little later, when I knew Rost better, I told him how surprised I had been at hearing pidgin from a blue-eyed man. He smiled, amused and interested himself in the phenomenon, but not especially pleased that he had been the one who exhibited it. It was not an effect he was striving for.

Rost is from Pennsylvania, born and raised. He first came to the Islands before the war, and settled in Kipahulu when the war was over. He loved the quiet in Kipahulu. "You don't see many roads like this on the mainland, do you?" he asked of the stony track beneath us. It was a road that would offend the sensibilities of many people back in

Pennsylvania; narrow, winding, and rutted, but Rost liked it.

I thought, as I rode along, about how these green islands and gentle people invade their invaders. Here, on Maui, was a tattooed Pennsylvania man talking pidgin, sitting beside a brown wife and grandson. It was the kind of transformation that happened in the South Seas, I knew, in Melville's and in Maugham's times, but not now, in our fiftieth state, a state with a city like Honolulu in it. Here was William Rost—and it cannot seem to him that he has been here long—with a dark wife at his side, and already a dark grandson.

William Rost was standing outside his house one evening, under his coco palms, watching the sky over the Pacific run through its last colors before somberness. His favorite dog walked up and nuzzled his hand. It was a three-legged dog, covered with scars from past fights with wild pigs. He had once been Rost's best hunting dog, Rost said as he scratched him. Now he was thirteen years old and crippled by pigs, but he could still hunt. Rost could

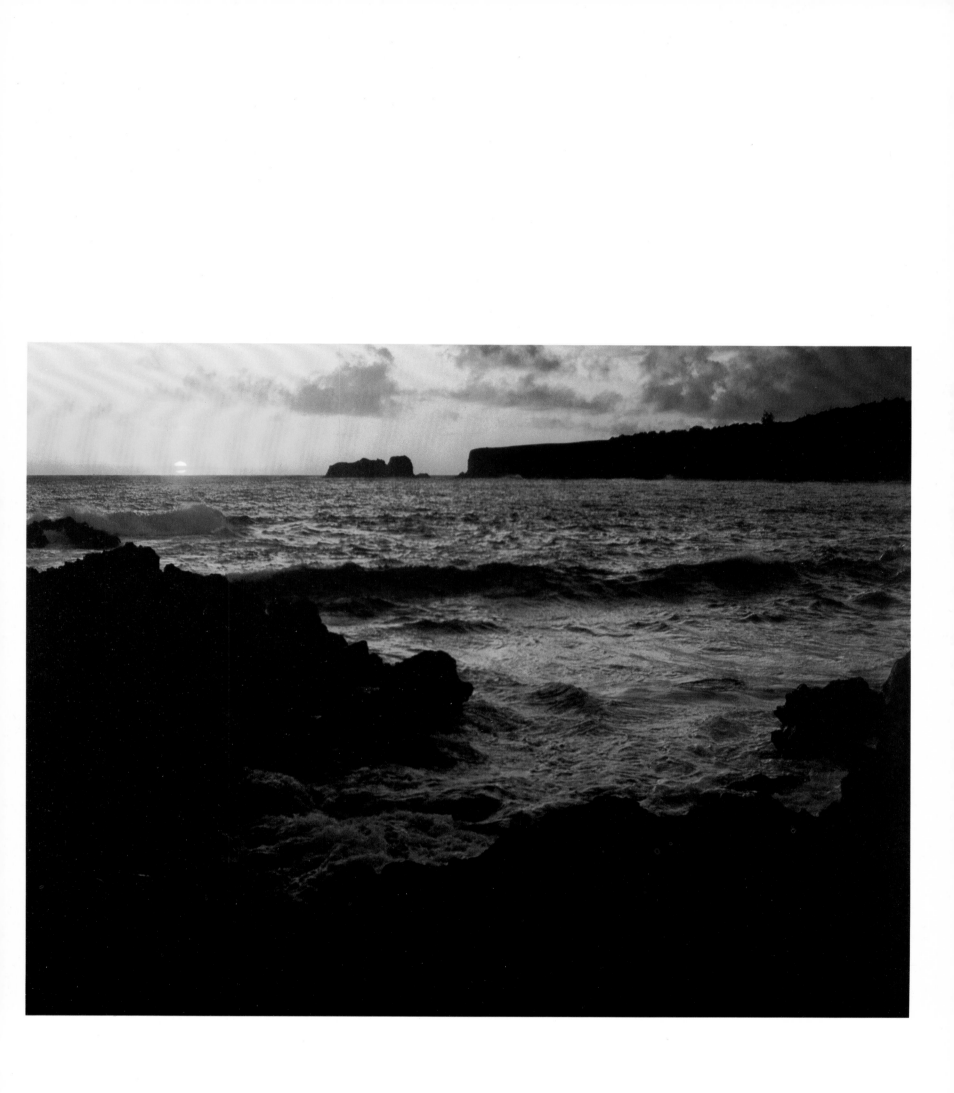

not let him go after pigs in the underbrush, but if the pig was in open pasture, the dog would do all right. I asked Rost if he and his dog liked fishing too, and he said he didn't go for it. "I'm a mountain man. Hunting, that's me," he said.

I liked to listen to Rost talk. There are strange mixtures of idiom in pidgin, and especially Rost's pidgin, that were always surprising. "Living's dear," he would say, with an inflection that sounded British to me, but a moment later would say, "Bime by," just as a Mark Twain Mississippi character would have. Sometimes his language had a stately sound ("For to buy flour") that was heightened by his refusal to use contractions ("That I do not know.")

Rost has never gone home again. He thinks about returning from time to time, and decides against it. It has been too long and his family would no longer know him, he says.

"My mother last saw me as a boy, and now . . ." He indicated himself with a small gesture of his hand. His lean face lined and his neck weathered from his years in the Hawaiian sun, his chin stubbled and grizzly. Like most Hawaiians of his age in Kipahulu, he was missing several teeth. ". . . she might drop dead," he said.

Rost does not want his son to go to the mainland, though Mrs. Rost urges it. Rost's son is married to a Hawaiian girl, and Rost worries about her on the mainland, for he has heard about the racial violence there. "Your wife is of a different race," he has warned his son. The violence distresses Rost. When he was in school in Pennsylvania, he says, he was in the same classroom with Negroes. Both boys and girls. They sat on benches in them days—on the same bench! He can't understand the trouble there now, and he has advised his son not to go.

In his mother's last letters she told Rost how everything had changed at home. There are highways and buildings where there were none before, and life is different. The prospect makes Rost uncomfortable, and he does not like to think of returning.

Happily, he never has to. He can stand outside his house on mild winter evenings, resting from his day's work for the County, and with his three-legged dog for company can watch, as he was watching the evening I last dropped by, while his son and daughter-in-law, bundled against what Hawaiians call the cold, load their fishing tackle and long bamboo poles into the station wagon and set out for a night's surf fishing, an enterprise the hunter and his dog can then shake their heads at.

The Kaiwis

The day after Thanksgiving Jack Kaiwi invited his friends to dinner. There was still turkey left, in spite of Jack's sixteen children and his one grandchild. The adults and older children ate first that evening, and the younger children waited in the next room and watched television. The large kitchen table was set with paper plates. There were canned peas and corn, rice, turkey, carrot sticks in a water glass, and pumpkin pie. The men drank beer and the women Nesbitts orange pop.

The kitchen was roomy. By the far door was a painting of a mountain lion that Jack had bought for the children for bow and arrow practice. The arrows were the kind with suction cups, Jack explained. There were no arrows in the lion at the moment. Tacked to the beams of the ceiling were several of the cocker spaniel paintings that you buy in variety stores, and against the near wall was a red starfish, made by Roberta Kaiwi from cowrie shells.

Everyone but Jack Lind and me was Catholic, and they all crossed themselves before beginning. Jack and I looked down at our plates as Helene Kaiwi delivered a benediction, not a word of which I could understand.

The dinner talk began immediately afterward. It started with the painted lion, and went from there to bow and arrow hunting. Jack Lind and Jack Kaiwi talked respectfully about the two archers who had come to Kipahulu several years before to hunt pigs. Then everyone talked about how wet it had been over the weekend, and Jack Kaiwi admitted how lazy he had been with the rain for an excuse.

Daisy and Helene talked about the Hawaiian chef at the Hana hotel. He was a great instinctive cook, they said, who had been traveling around lately, learning more about his trade. He had knocked the eyes out of the haoles at the hotel with his Thanksgiving creations. His most ingenious was a salad, lit from beneath, that looked like an erupting volcano. You had to admit, Daisy said, that Hawaiians know how to put on a show.

When the parents had finished eating, the children came in and began. After this second sitting had finished, the Kaiwi daughters cleared the table. The grown Linds and Kaiwis stayed in the kitchen to play cribbage, and everyone else went into the living room to watch television.

The living room was dark. There were more wall reliefs made of sea shells. There was a felt tapestry of a religious subject on one wall, several small mounted birds, a set of goat horns, and a Christ over the door. All sixteen Kaiwi children, and several of their friends were there, and the room was full of small Hawaiians. There were three sofas, two of them made up as beds, and tonight they were crowded. There was a pallet on the floor on which the youngest children would later sleep, and on which they now sat, watching. The pallet was long, and it must have slept seven or eight Kaiwis.

The television stood in a corner on a strange pedestal— a wooden, ziggurat-shaped thing, its original purpose impossible to determine. On top of the set was a Virgin, and beside the Virgin was a dark wooden sculpture that looked child-made and pagan, but the light was dim and it may have been something less mysterious. Above the Virgin, where the walls met in the corner, hung the great polished shell of a Pacific green turtle. It all made for a strange altar.

The childrens' faces were lit partly by the television, and partly by the light from the kitchen, where the cribbage game went on. The faces were not lit brightly enough to tell which of the children belonged to the two sets of twins, or which of the children were best looking. They all looked handsome.

First "Lucy" came on, and then "Ensign Pulver," a movie that no one particularly enjoyed. We waited it out, though, because wrestling from Honolulu came next.

Leroy Kaiwi and Duffy Lind were good friends and sat together watching. Occasionally they wrestled with each other absent-mindedly. When they weren't wrestling Leroy leaned against Duffy's legs and watched the screen. They were both about sixteen, and were natural in a kind of intimacy that boys their age in less tropic and more anxious climes would avoid. The little Kaiwi girls were forever getting up and leaving the room on some mission, and would proudly say, "Excuse me," as they passed.

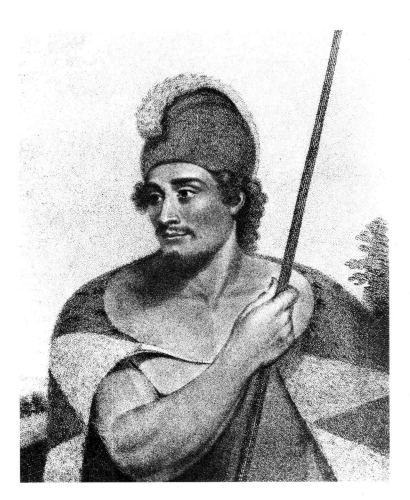

On Saturdays many Kipahulu men like to go pig hunting, and the older Kaiwi boys are among them. One Saturday morning of the rainy season, two of the Kaiwis decided to go. Paul Kaiwi brought a short, single-shot .22 in an olive-drab case. His little brother Earl brought a machete. He called it a bolo knife, as they do in the Philippines, and he carried it with some pride. Earl had a bad cold, but he was anxious to go along. He was wearing a blue cub scout's shirt with a wolf badge and three achievement arrows. The insignia had been torn from the shoulder, and had left a patch of darker blue. The shirt was untucked, and Earl was sniffling.

Earl Kaiwi was in the eighth grade. He was slighter and fairer than Paul, and showed more clearly that the Kaiwis have some Oriental blood. Paul himself is swarthy and his hair is curly. For him, as he says, "the Chinese doesn't pull."

The brothers parked a ranch jeep in their backyard and collected the hunting dogs. There were several old cars in the yard, two or three of which looked as if they might run. The two dogs that were new to hunting, and not anxious to begin learning, took refuge under the cars. Paul dragged the first out from under a battered, green Model-A truck with bald tires. The dog was miserable, and his protest sounded desperate as he came unwillingly into sight, snapping at the rope leash that was dragging him. Paul was training him for a friend for twenty-five dollars, and the dog had gone hunting only twice before. Paul took him to the jeep, and, while Earl held him there, Paul went after the other young dog. As he lifted this one in his arms, it gave a very dismal little cry. In contrast the lead dog, who was part airedale and an experienced hunter, came willingly, as did two other old dogs, and they all started up to the forest.

The jeep bounced up the high wet pasture. Paul stopped at each pasture gate, opened it, then closed it behind him, and continued on. Earl, sitting in the back and holding the novice dogs, turned from time to time and watched the misty pillars of rain squalls moving below on the gray plane of the Pacific. The young dogs were restless, and twice Paul warned his younger brother not to let them jump out. Earl broke up two dog fights, and the jeep, slowing almost to a stop where the trail was bad, speeding up where the slope was gentler, arrived at the edge of the guava forest.

Just as the jeep stopped, rain started falling. The brothers ran to the shelter of the guavas. Paul hung the rifle case from a guava branch and stood to wait the rain out. Suddenly, it began to come down harder. The guava canopy was poor protection, and the brothers ran back to the jeep. They found some empty feed bags in the back, tore them open, and squatting in the lee of the jeep, held the bags over their heads. They sat there for twenty minutes, watching the rain fall or watching their feet. They said little, for no one talks much when he's trying to keep out of the rain, and young Hawaiians talk very little anyway. The brothers fell into a rain trance.

The dogs looked very bleak with the water running off them. They waited in the open for the hunt to begin and looked from time to time into their masters' faces. Every once in a while one would shake himself, and be roundly cursed and threatened for it.

When the rain let up, Paul unleashed the airedale. The dog bolted, and entered the forest accelerating. The brothers followed, more slowly. The other dogs, whom Paul calls "grabbers," were not so fit as the airedale, a "trailer," who could run all day. The grabbers stayed with the hunters, waiting for the trailer to pick up the scent.

The forest was pleasant to walk in. The ferns and fungi, and the black earth, were washed by the storm. The rain brought out the smell of guavas lying on the ground, and the air was sweet with it. The hunting was leisurely as the brothers stopped often to listen for the airedale's bark. In the silences, when the brothers strained to hear any distant sound, the reality of the forest obtruded on them. Sound traveled better in the forest when it was wet. The brothers could hear all the tickings and tiny sounds of the forest's life. In the places where they paused and listened, the dripping forest came into focus for them. Earl thought he heard the airedale bark. Paul, with older, or perhaps less imaginative ears, did not hear it, and after two hours the brothers left the dog to his pursuits and went home.

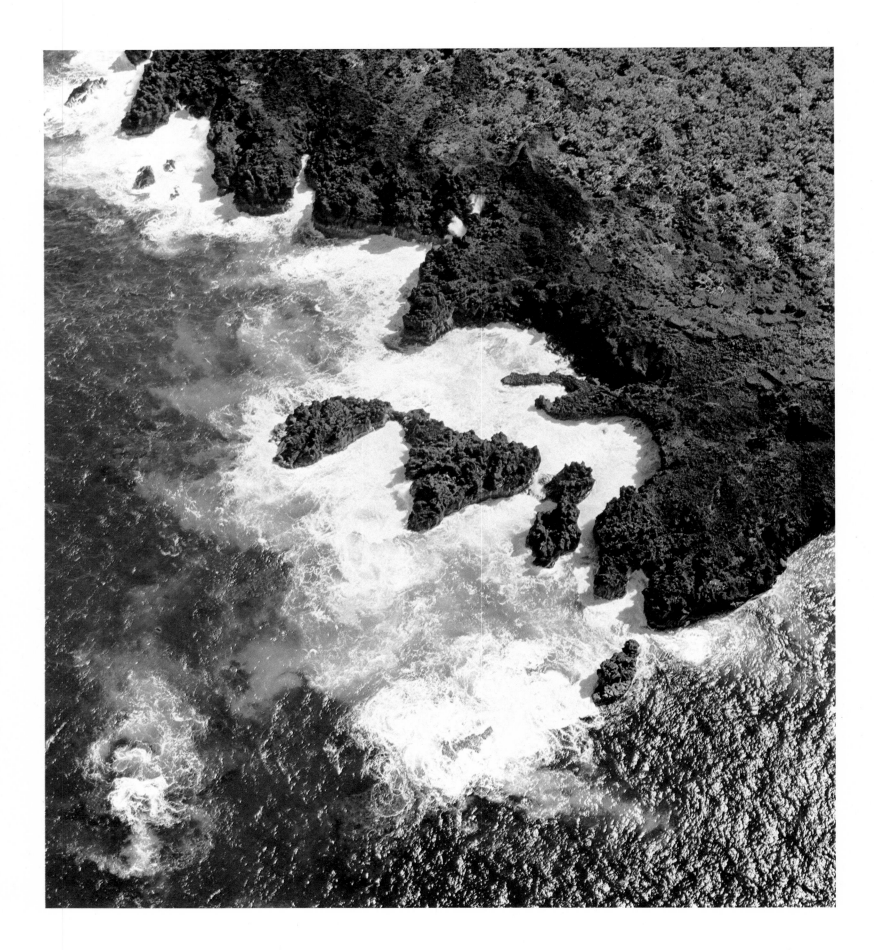

Pelipe Bernabe

The repair shed at Kipahulu Ranch is an open building with a hard earth floor. Pigeons perch on its corrugated roof, and a land breeze from the slopes of Haleakala blows in through the back. There is usually a jeep there undergoing repairs, and a modest assortment of power tools lies about.

In the daytime Pelipe Bernabe sits in the shed and, leaning on his cane, watches the men work. He is a small brown man, so old that it is hard to tell what his ancestry is. He could be Hawaiian, or he could be Filipino, which seems more likely from his name. He is so insubstantial a presence that the men work and talk as if he weren't there. They move and laugh around him, and he watches with interest. He leans on his cane and mutely supervises, peering hard at the engine being worked over, or craning his neck to watch the approach of a wrench in Jack Kaiwi's hand. He seems always on the verge of giving instructions, but never does.

I turned once to see his very clear eyes regarding me intently, but the moment our eyes met he looked away.

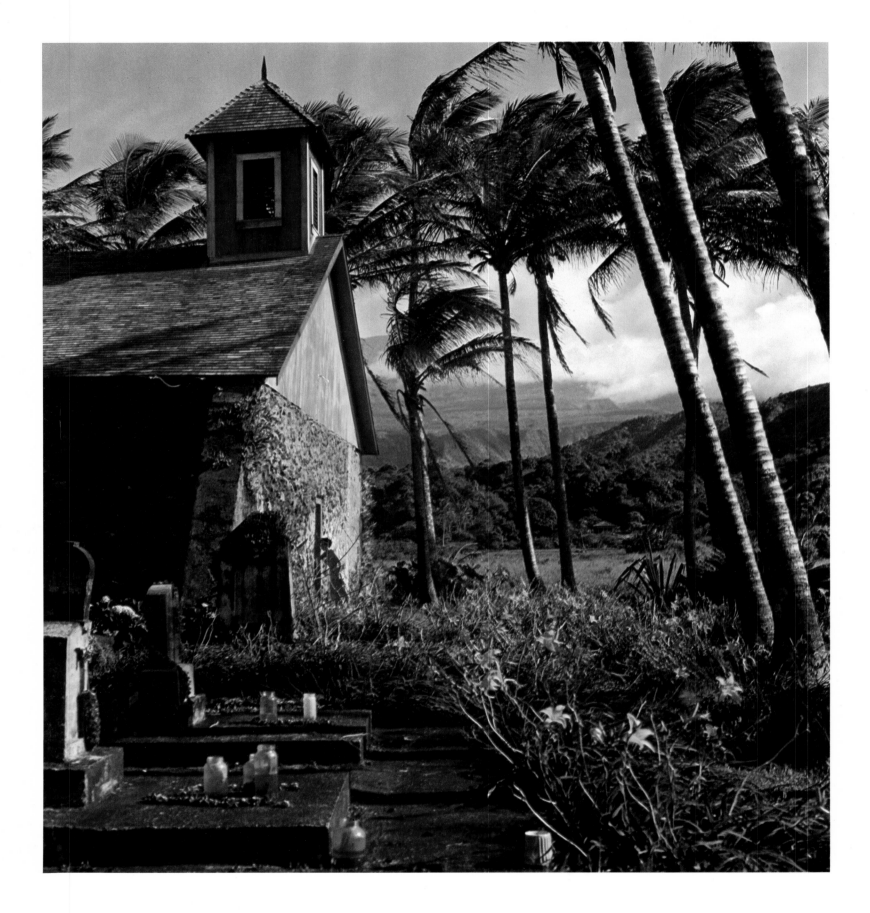

Nick Soon

For forty years Nick Soon has run the store at Kaupo. Nick is seventy-five years old but looks much younger. His store looks its age; a building of weathered wood and very small windows facing the sea. There is a porch, bare usually except for a box or two of empty pop bottles. There is a set of double doors, painted yellow a long time ago, and a small sign above that reads "Kaupo Store." If Nick Soon himself shows his years, it is in his limbs. His arms and hands are so frail that I had a little shock as I shook hands with him, and instantly eased my pressure, hoping I hadn't hurt anything. Nick's face is still young, his eyes shrewd and quick.

Nick Soon's father owned several Chinese stores on Maui, of which the Kaupo store was one, and he had the opium concession for the entire island, according to a local story. Nick himself is not so dedicated a businessman, but he has skills that compensate. It is locally agreed that Nick Soon is a mechanical genius. Nick built the first generator on East Maui, and assembled or imported the first Model T's. For years his cars plied the short road from the Kaupo dock to Kaupo Village, filled with store goods and with Hawaiians along for the ride. Nick, with his electricity, cars, model planes, and his curiosity, introduced his part of the Maui coast to the Age of the Machine.

The day we dropped by his store, Nick was getting settled, having just returned from a trip to Tahiti and Samoa. He had a hundred relatives in Tahiti, he told us. One of them, a bright young man only forty-three-years old, was a millionaire.

Nick had liked Tahiti and Samoa, but found those places backward. Samoa was far behind Hawaii, and Tahiti was about twenty years behind. If you don't speak French or Chinese you are finished in Tahiti, Nick told us. It had taken Nick a while to remember his Chinese. For forty years he had spoken only Hawaiian to the Kaupo cowboys who came to his store, and English to outsiders. Fortunately the Chinese dialect spoken in Tahiti had been his own.

The Tahitians don't understand Hawaiian, he said, and this seemed to annoy him. When I asked if any of the words were the same, he drew a notebook from his pocket, and read a long list of the words he had found that were common to both languages.

As he came to the end of his list, Nick's manner, which is always curt and stiff, became more so. He had been closed when we arrived and had stopped what he was doing to open for us. He was beginning to regret it. We paid for the orange pop we were drinking, thanked him and said good-bye. He went back to sorting the six hundred photographs he had taken on his Polynesian trip—very ordinary photographs, I am told, most of them of people standing awkwardly in front of buildings.

Nick Soon is no longer seriously in the store business. He is closed much of the time, and his shelves are almost empty. The Hawaiian cowboys and all the gay Hawaiian syllables that once filled his store no longer fill it. Habit is strong in Nick Soon, however, and he is not quite ready to retire.

The busy plantation days that Nick photographed and was a part of ended in the twenties, and since then things have been slowing down on the Kipahulu coast. Perhaps the quiet bothers him, for he is contemplating another trip to Tahiti.

A rough road now connects the Kaupo Store with Hana and the rest of Maui, and Nick Soon no longer gets his goods by sea. The old road to his landing, winding around black lava pinnacles and steeply down to the water, the road that was once so intimately known to his Model T, is now little traveled—by a lost steer perhaps, or, as on at least one afternoon, by a brown fisherman, his long pole on his shoulder, trudging home from the sea.

The Land

In Kipahulu, on a promontory above the sea, are the remains of a great temple. Much of the temple's length is buried under the earth swell of the promontory, but one end lies open to the sky and gives an idea of the temple's original size. The exposed part is one hundred feet high and massive, built of black lava stones that are very regular in their size and roundness. The steep slant of the temple wall, though interrupted in many places by the grass that has pushed out between the stones, is still impressive. The top of the temple, where not overgrown, is still remarkably flat. There is a certain rock on the top that lifted aside reveals a narrow crack, and from the crack, as you can feel if you put your cheek to it, blows a cool air current. The current hints at rooms or passages below, but there has been no serious excavation and no one knows.

There are many *heiaus*, or temples, on East Maui, for its coast was once one of the most populous in the Islands. Maui's green slopes and offshore waters once fed many more people than they do in our poorer times, and the people then were dedicated builders. Their few descendants on this coast today are simpler architects, with no instinct for the heavy monuments of the past. They do not regard the old architecture as part of their history, and feel no pride or responsibility for it. When asked about the heiaus, many Hawaiians still answer, with little interest, "The *menehunes* did that." The little people. What reasonable man, and who but supernatural folk, could be concerned with such undertakings?

Today the Hawaiians in Kipahulu are Catholic, and a quarter of a mile from the heiau, St. Paul's church now stands. On Saturdays the residents go to Mass there, for the priest must travel about the island, and on Sundays he is elsewhere. The steeple of St. Paul's is only thirty feet high, and the cross on top is a simple one fashioned from iron pipe. The church is painted a bright Easter-egg blue. It is a very pretty color, believe it or not, set as it is against the green of pasture and of high distant forest. There are carefully tended red flowers under the windows, and young palms above the corrugated iron roof. The windows are always open, even when church is not in service, and the air inside is always fresh. After the high stark mounds of the old religion, St. Paul's seems very innocent. The old priests, hard and grim men, conductors of human sacrifice, would disapprove. But the old priests are dead, and for several hundred years the Maui rain has been falling on their temple stones, the grass rising between and rolling those stones aside.

One hundred yards down the road from St. Paul's church are the ruins of a sugar mill. The mill's low building is overgrown and its original shape undeterminable, but its single tall concrete chimney, cracked but handsome, still rises from the grass. The heavy iron doors of the boiler are still accessible. One of them has rusted shut, but the other swings free. The door opens, a rude intrusion, on banyan roots that have grown down through the flue and are carrying on their work in the dark where mill fires once burned. The boiler is at the very heart of the hill, yet the roots have penetrated. They must then have insinuated themselves through every part of the mill, and be working in every part at its overthrow. The mill still stands, but disuse has brought it an anonymity. The chimney should be the most impressive structure around, but, dehumanized now and without function, its spirit has departed and it does not catch the eye. The chimney is at the edge of a bull pasture, and the bulls grazing under it, though only mild Herefords, attract more attention.

The Kipahulu mill, and the old bridges that served it, are vestiges of the plantation days of East Maui, days when this coast was busier and more populous, days of night trucks and Negro camps, of Chinese camps, cane fires, and the heat of human endeavor. The simple concrete bridges, with dates of construction; 1912, 1914, 1916, chiseled on them in an old calligraphy, are somber and patinaed now, their surfaces as satisfactory to moss as forest stones. They have not echoed to the passage of cane trucks for a generation, and in this new age are quiet.

Banyan tree, Kipahulu Churchyard

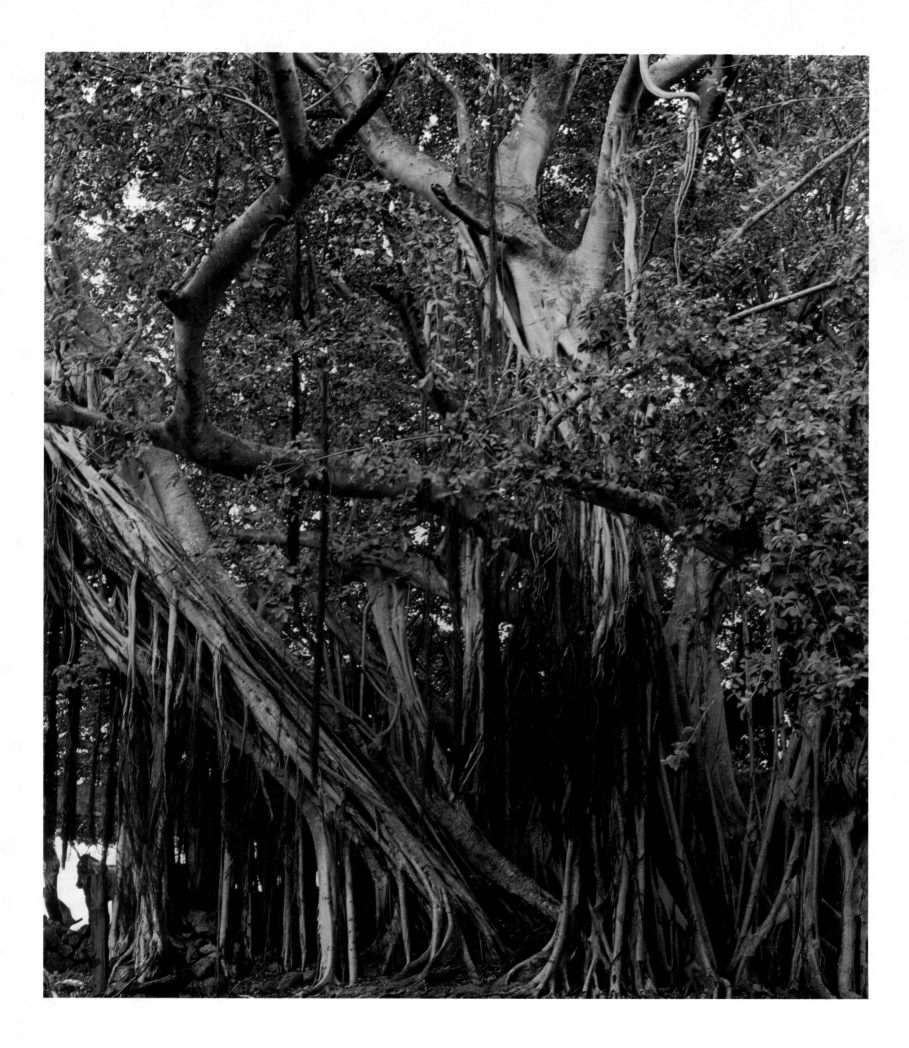

At the point where the path from the Kipahulu heiau meets the Kipahulu road, on *makai* side of the road, is a low stone wall. Whatever there is that does not love a wall has not loved this one, and has tumbled and interrupted it in several places. Beyond the wall, all but lost in a thick forest of palms, is an abandoned house. It is possible to walk past the house several times without seeing it, for the same forces at work on the wall have obscured the house. It has tilted, through some movement of the earth or defect in design, at a sharp angle to its old foundation. Green vines climb its walls and yellow flowers grow out over its roof. Only the dark and empty windows catch the eye.

The house is inviting, as most dead houses are, but inaccessible. The tumbled lava wall encloses what may once have been a garden but is now wildly overgrown and impassible without a machete.

Whether the house dates from plantation times or later—what its history is—is hard to say. Whenever I passed it, though, it reminded me in a forceful way that the Rome of this coast is past, its history over. The great days of the plantations, days when this air was full with the palpable raw sweetness of cane, and the Polynesian days when thousands lived here, built temples, fought each other, hunted these forests and fished these inlets—the days when this coast had a future—are done. Yet each time I saw the house, vague in the palm shadows, I had to correct a first brief impression that it was a woman and wore yellow flowers in its hair. The coast of East Maui, if past its Rome, is returning to its Eden.

False kamani leaves

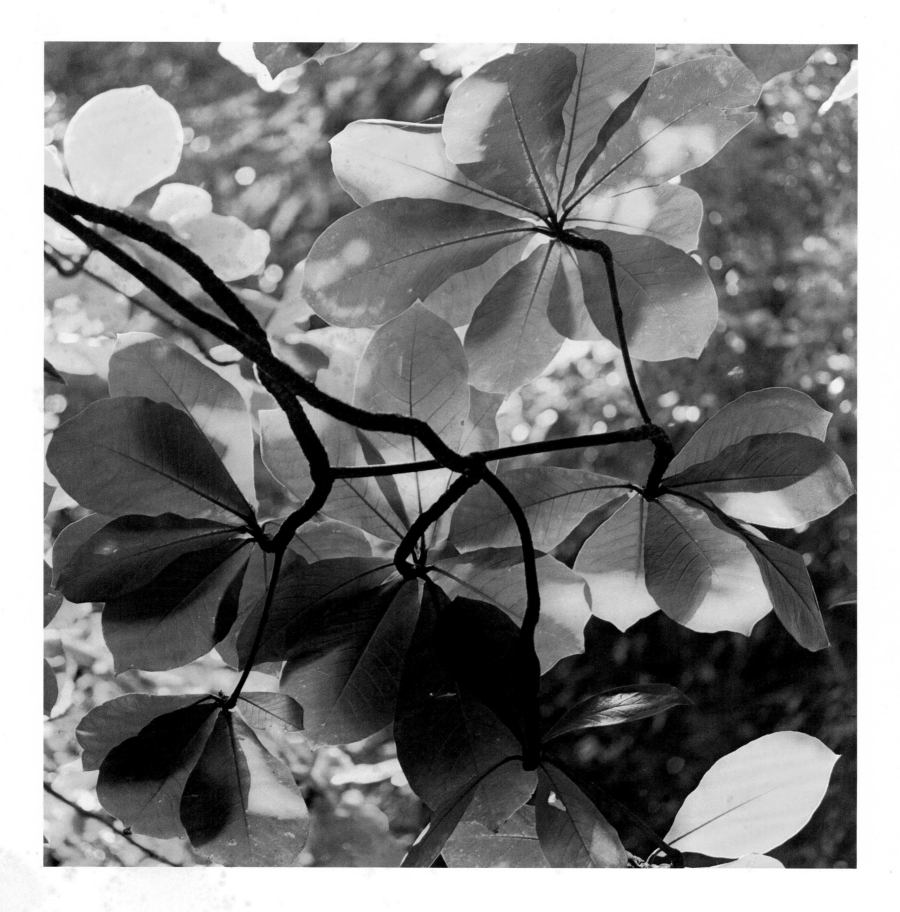

Friends of the Earth in the United States, and sister organizations of the same name in other countries, are working for the preservation, restoration, and more rational use of the earth. We urge people to make more intensive use of the branches of government that society has set up for itself. Within the limits of support given us, we try to represent the public's interest in the environment before administrative and legislative bodies and in court. We add to, and need, the diversity of the conservation front in its vital effort to build greater respect for the earth and its living resources, including man.

We lobby for this idea. We work closely with our sister organizations abroad, and with new and old conservation organizations here and abroad that have saved so much for all of us to work for.

We publish—books, like this, and in smaller format—because of our belief in the power of the book and also to help support ourselves. Our environmental newspaper is "Not Man Apart."

If the public press is the fourth estate, perhaps we are the fifth. We speak out for you; we invite your support.

Friends of the Earth Foundation, also in San Francisco, supports the work of Friends of the Earth and organizations like it with projects in litigation and in scientific research, literature, and education.

Publisher's Note: The book is set in Centaur and Arrighi by Mackenzie & Harris Inc., San Francisco. It was lithographed and bound by Arnoldo Mondadori Editore, Verona, on coated paper made by Cartiera Celdit and Bamberger Kaliko Fabrik. The design is by David Brower. The Layout is by Kenneth Brower.

Endpaper photograph: False Kamani leaves, by Robert Wenkam.

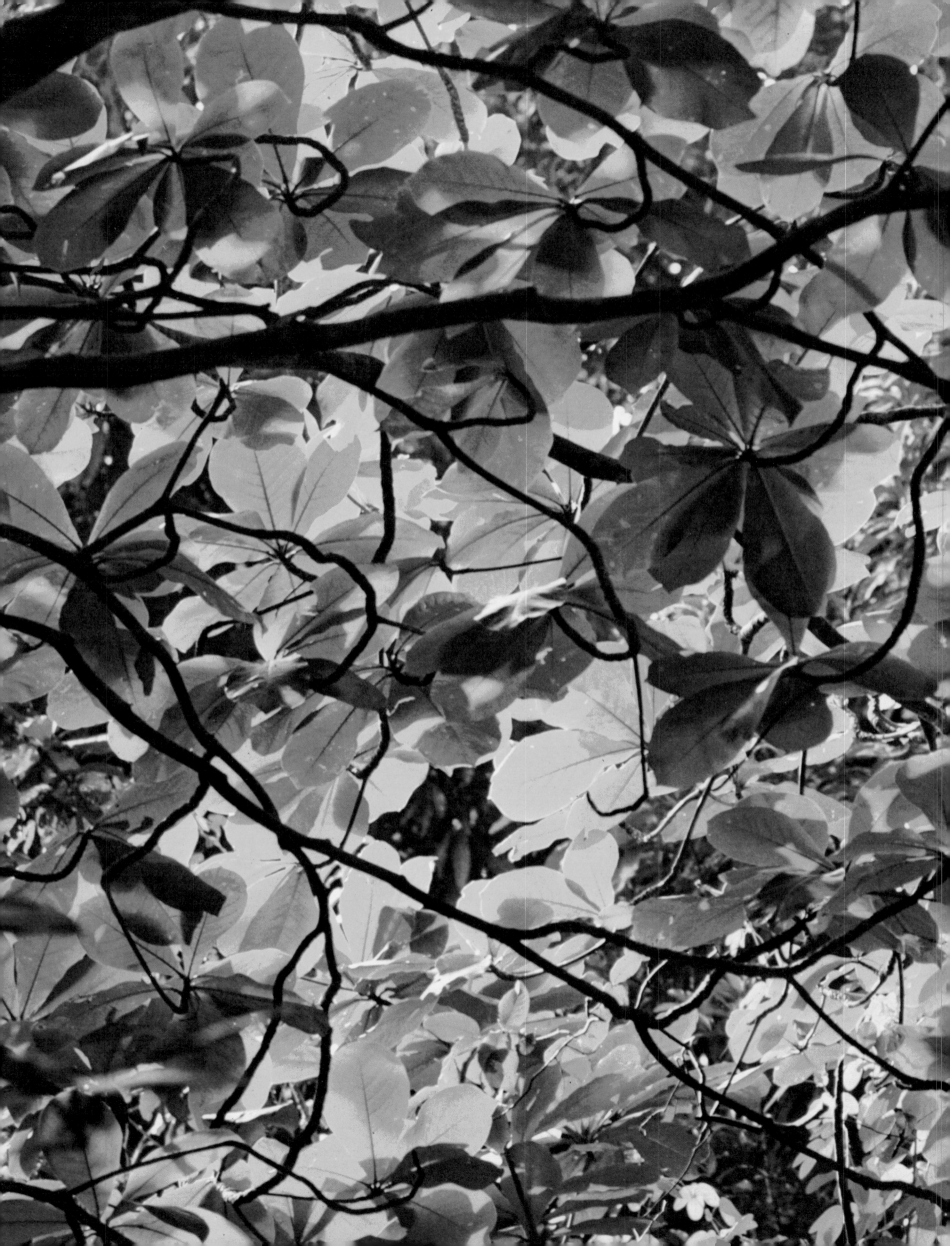